Informed: The Art of Preparing Athletes

Paul Gamble PhD

Informed: The Art of the Science of Preparing Athletes

First published February 2018 by Informed in Sport, Vancouver, Canada.

ISBN (e-book): 978-1-7752186-1-6

ISBN (paperback): 978-1-7752186-0-9

Table of Contents

Table of Figures

Foreword

"Making systems work… is the great task of our generation as a whole. In every field, knowledge has exploded, but it has brought complexity, it has brought specialization. And we've come to a place where we have no choice but to recognize, as individualistic as we want to be, complexity requires group success. We all need to be pit crews now."

– Atul Gawande

The world of high performance sport is a cacophony of information, new technology and highly specialized personnel. Add to this the silos, egos and professional turf battles and you have many challenges to building a successful team in support of elite athletes. Many of us think we should be the race car driver; in reality, we are the pit crew. We are human beings, working in close relation to one another, not independently.

While evidenced-based practices and data collection are important, it is the traits of critical thinking, humility, reflection and careful decision making are the foundation for long-term success and a culture of excellence. These are often referred to as "soft skills" – skills that are not generally addressed in formal academic preparation, and areas that are outside traditional sport science areas of biomechanics, physiology and biochemistry. Pursuit and mastery of these "soft" skills are an essential part of the "art" behind any successful coach or sports medicine practitioner who is a part of a performance team.

In his latest book, *Informed: The Art of the Science of Preparing Athletes*, Paul Gamble defines what it means to be an informed practitioner, coach and athlete, and in the process provides a compass for us all to navigate the vast world that is high performance sport. To be informed is to develop a frame of reference and a body of experience to effectively curate and apply the information presented to us by sport science. To be effective, we must also seek out and develop the leadership, communication and teaching skills to build relationships with athletes, and to seamlessly integrate with other members of the performance team. In the real world, effective practice is contingent on our ability to successfully apply what we know in real-time, to real situations.

This is not a textbook. Having written multiple textbooks on team and individual sport preparation, Paul steps behind the physical, technical and tactical to shed light on the 'human' part of human performance. This new offering is a guidebook to help us develop our own "reflective practice with teeth." It is witty, candid and doesn't pretend to have all the answers. After all, more often than not, the answer is "it depends."

Human performance is messy, complicated and imperfect. And while we plan, we must be agile and ready to adapt, improvise and overcome the anxiety that comes with deviating from our carefully constructed plan, or the fact "that's the way we've always done it before." We must also consider context, because without context, any one training plan or rehabilitation protocol is effectively "without teeth."

There are times when we must break with tradition and the inertia of old practice patterns to successfully respond to the situation before us and to grow as coaches and practitioners. In my own professional journey, I have endeavoured to see the worlds of strength and conditioning and rehabilitation with different eyes. I have tried to think outside the squat rack and the khaki pants, to break down the silos and find what unites these two distinct, often divisive, professional worlds and mindsets. I have had the privilege of working in both worlds, and the opportunity to collaborate and share my experiences and reflections with my peers. It is only through sharing, discussion and reflection that we have the potential to become better informed and more capable professionals.

This book provides a framework for all human performance professionals, novice and experienced, to come together, reflect and grow. We should aspire to truly be informed, not just educated. To that end we must view things with a healthy skepticism, a broadened perspective and a deeper understanding of the process behind developing elite athletes.

Each chapter in this book offers a pit stop in support of developing your own reflective practice. You will come away not only inspired to raise the bar in your own little corner of the sporting world, but also equipped with practical tools and ideas to help you survive the fire hose of information that our world of electronic connection brings us on a daily basis.

Tracy Fober, Physical Therapist and Strength Coach, US Ski and Snowboard Association. Park City, UT. January 2018.

Preface

This book came about via a somewhat circuitous route. In late 2015 I set up an online platform (informedinsport.com) to share ideas and content on topical subjects and recurring themes from my discussions with colleagues, peers, and practitioners under my mentorship. My intention was to pass on some of the experience gained from working with outstanding coaches, practitioners and athletes over a number of years across a variety of sports. My intended audience from the outset was therefore coaches, practitioners, and athletes themselves. The Informed Blog has been well received and some readers have been kind enough to offer feedback, including the suggestion that the content might make a good book. Hence many of the chapters to follow are developed from the original content which began its life as the Informed Blog. Regular readers of the Informed Blog will also find chapters with 'all new' content on themes not shared previously.

To explain the title, there is an art to translating what empirical evidence is available in the sports science literature and applying this information in practice with 'live' athletes. By their nature, athletes represent a 'special population'. Moreover as a population elite athletes have not been extensively studied. As such, there is always a need to bridge the gap between textbook learning and the real-life conditions encountered when working with athletes. This involves a great deal of interpretation, understanding of context, and nuance to translate the limited information that exists in order to inform practice. No part of this process is customarily covered in a textbook or research publication.

Indeed many of the areas we delve into in the chapters that follow are not generally catered for in any meaningful way within the formal learning pathways that exist for applied practitioners in sports science and sports medicine. So in addition to those currently working in sport, this book is also for students of these domains; essentially, those who aspire to become the next generation of coaches, practitioners and perhaps athletes.

"Where is the wisdom we have lost in knowledge? Where is the knowledge we have lost in information?"

– T.S. Eliot

In this era of connectivity there is unprecedented access to information. The challenge for those who wish to be informed becomes one of navigating these seas of information, and attempting to derive meaning. The task of separating signal from noise has become extremely challenging, as the level of noise in the social media and Information Age has reached such a level. Whilst the content in each chapter includes citations to steer the reader to the relevant literature on each topic, it is nevertheless these higher order skills of critical reasoning, problem-solving, and decision-making that are the real focus.

Reflecting its inception, this book is a departure from the previous textbooks I have written. Returning once more to the title, there is art in the experiential wisdom that informs the science of preparing athletes. Ultimately to effectively apply the knowledge acquired from books and other resources requires the frame of reference to do so.

"Words without experience are meaningless."

— Vladimir Nabokov

Throughout the chapters that follow I have tried to provide examples from my own journey and experiences of working in elite sport that feature in the chapters. Equally, I readily acknowledge that the perspectives shared on different topics in the book are coloured by my own set of experiences and influences.

"Spoon feeding in the long run teaches us nothing but the shape of the spoon"

E.M. Forster

In order to reflect reality, any resource on coaching must also recognise complexity. I have been conscious to avoid proposing facile answers to complex questions. There are no universal solutions; it all depends upon the context of the situation. The importance of context is an important theme that recurs throughout this book. Ultimately it is incumbent upon the reader to determine how this information applies to their own environment and the individual athletes concerned.

Clearly when writing any resource that concerns preparing athletes it is important to recognise that we are dealing with humans. Whatever the discipline concerned, there is very little certainty with the outcome when working with such complex adaptive systems. The content that follows aims to reconcile this idea. To find a way forward we must embrace the uncertainty to be adaptive in our approach. By definition this does not lend itself to a cookie-cutter approach. Rather, my aim is to equip the reader with an understanding of governing principles and an appreciation of the relevant parameters to apply them to the situation at hand.

Finally, whatever the discipline, ultimately effective practice is contingent upon our interaction with the athlete. The human interaction element of coaching and applied practice is a major theme of this book, and we will delve into the realms of leadership, pedagogy, skill refinement, and mental skills. The ultimate test of the coach is what happens when they are not present: the critical importance of developing autonomy, and the role of the athlete in the process is emphasised throughout the chapters that follow.

Acknowledgements

I would first like to acknowledge those individuals I have mentored and the colleagues and peers in different corners the globe who took part in the discussions which were the genesis of the ideas and themes that feature in the chapters that follow.

Each of the athletes I have been fortunate to work with during my career to date has taught me something about what it is to be a coach, and added to my understanding of the dynamics and multiple facets of the processes of physical and athletic preparation. It remains a privilege, and I continue to be grateful for the ongoing lessons.

I would like to recognise my father Steve as the person who has taught me more about leadership, managing teams, and working with humans than anybody.

Finally, I would like to dedicate this book to my wife, Sian. A central theme in this book is that the crucial first step to being a good coach and practitioner is to be a good human; the miracle of being your other half gives my life meaning, and drives me to be a better man. I aspire to one day prove myself worthy…

Part One: For the Practitioner

Section One – Communicating and Guiding

Cultivating Coaching Craft

As practitioners we are all coaches. Irrespective of what sub-discipline a practitioner may operate within, there is inevitably some element of instruction involved. Ultimately, the knowledge of the coach or practitioner is of limited value without this ability to express and convey the relevant information. A key facet of the art of coaching is therefore communicating information in a way that the athlete is able to understand. Coaching must also be delivered in a way that the athlete can process effectively. Finally, the feedback and instruction needs to be distilled into actionable steps to enable the athlete to effect the necessary changes and produce the desired outcome. In this chapter we will explore each of these themes.

THERE ARE ALWAYS TWO COACHES...

Is it important to commence with the understanding that, in addition to our voice, inside the head of the athlete there is also the voice of the athlete's own 'inner coach'.

With this realisation we can begin to account for this inner voice, and to harness it. We can also try to capture some of the athlete's internal coaching process. As part of the athlete's daily diary process we can ask them to note down what cues, mental images, or other triggers they found effective and helpful to executing the desired skill. It should be explicit that this should include any self-generated 'internal cues', images, or other representations of the skill that they come up with themselves, as well as any instruction we deliver.

VERIFYING MESSAGE RECEIVED...

Inevitably there is some degree of distortion between what is said and what is heard by the athlete. These considerations include not only the athlete's interpretation of the instruction given, but even what particular words they latch onto.

It is often revealing to ask the athlete what they understood or what they heard from the instruction given. Often it is apparent that there is some discrepancy between what was said and what message was received.

We also need to acknowledge legacy effects resulting from previous exposure to other coaches, and consider how this prior experience may have shaped the athlete's perception and understanding. Unless the athlete is a complete novice, there will inevitably be some preconceptions to unpack.

FINDING THE KEY FOR THE ATHLETE...

Even when the technical model and idea to present to the athlete is the same, the method that proves effective for communicating this information to each individual can differ markedly.

Hence the challenge that faces the coach is finding the particular word or cue that resonates with the particular individual. What every coach aims for is that illuminating 'light bulb' moment when the message becomes meaningful to the athlete.

The route by which we arrive at this moment will differ for each athlete. The method of teaching that works for the majority will not work for all; it is clearly critical to accept this and prepare accordingly. To this end, having a broad and diverse playbook and an array of methods at your disposal is clearly beneficial.

Equally, a shotgun approach of throwing a variety of cues and methods of communicating all in one go can be baffling; and even if the athlete does pick up the relevant information it is very difficult in this situation to have a clear idea which cue or method proved effective. Building an understanding of the athlete and getting a sense of which cues and methods to select is therefore critical, not least for the ongoing discovery process and associated learning on the part of the coach.

Nevertheless, finding what is effective for different individuals is ultimately a trial and error process. With experience of communicating different messages to a variety of individuals a coach will acquire a growing playbook of cues and methods they have found to be effective, which are able to draw from.

PAINTING MENTAL PICTURES...

When it comes to coaching movement and technique, the information to be conveyed to the athlete is often in the form of concepts and quite abstract ideas. Often the quest is to conjure a visual depiction or a moving image in the mind of the athlete that captures the essence of what you are trying to convey. The use of analogies can be very useful here.

Other times it is a feeling that you are looking to capture. Simply manually putting the athlete in the posture you want can be very effective. Using tactile cues or describing the feel of the movement can also provide rich information that the athlete can readily apply. Ultimately our aim is that the athlete is provided with an accurate internal representation of the movement or skill we want them to perform.

Clearly this is however reliant on the coach or practitioner having an intimate understanding of the 'feel' of the movement in order that they are able to convey this information to the athlete. This does not necessarily mean that the coach must have been an elite performer themselves; it merely requires that the coach is willing to practice these movements on a regular basis in order that they are able to readily recall the sensations involved.

METHODS OF DELIVERY...

Relevant information can be conveyed by the coach in a variety of ways. This might be in the form of explicit instructions, or a detailed description of the skill or movement. Other information can also be delivered verbally, such as key themes, examples, and analogies. The language we choose is clearly important to express both meaning and desired emphasis. We can also use sounds to convey this information.

There are also a variety of non-verbal methods for providing instruction. Demonstration is perhaps the most common and well established forms of non-verbal instruction. The natural process of how we acquire new motor skills is for the learner to 'model' what they observe from those around them.

Clearly from this viewpoint, it would appear critical that the coach is able to demonstrate correct technique. Certainly this is a good test for any practitioner [1]. Many times when you are describing a particular movement to an athlete their response will be: 'show me'. More coaches and practitioners need to invest the necessary practice time to acquire the necessary mastery of the particular athletic skill to allow them to demonstrate with competence and thereby coach effectively.

That said, there are a growing number of tools available to the coach with the different resources such as YouTube that are readily available online that may provide a substitute for 'live' demonstration. Athletes are often highly adept at modelling movement behaviour from what they observe from video.

Similarly smart devices and related technology can be a great tool to inform and facilitate 'self-modelling'. Providing visual feedback in the form of video of the athlete themselves performing can be a very effective tool to augment other instruction provided.

One important consideration is that as coaches we are not dependent on any one coaching tool or method of delivery. We should aim to become adept with the full range of communication methods and modes of delivering information and feedback. The particular selection or blend will depend on the situation and the constraints of the environment, and what we find works best for the athlete.

THE JOURNEY...

As this discussion illustrates, it is not sufficient for the coach to have a detailed understanding of technique or technical model (albeit this is a necessary starting point!). The goal is to find the right message in the right manner of communicating the particular idea in a way that conveys the relevant information to the mind of the athlete. This comprises a host of different skills and experiential learning on the part of the coach or practitioner.

The process of acquiring these skills involves time spent coaching a mix of athletes at different stages of development, ideally in different environments and even different sports, a willingness to be innovative, and a commitment to reflective learning to get the most out of these experiences. Ultimately, this journey has no end point – even the best and most experienced coaches in the world are continually learning from each experience with a new athlete, adding to their playbook, and refining their approach.

Considered Coaching – When and How to Steer Athletes' Learning

I n the previous chapter we have spoken about the art of coaching and the power of well-chosen words. Regardless of what discipline a practitioner is working in (physical preparation, sports injury, coaching) there will be an element of coaching the athlete to perform movement. Coaching is integral to physical preparation, athletic development, injury rehabilitation, and essentially all aspects of working in sport. Becoming aware of the central tenets of skill acquisition and related considerations is a critical starting point when seeking to convey information to more effectively assist the learning process. The objective of this chapter is therefore to allow the practitioner to make the switch in mind-set from 'instruction' as being a process where the athlete is a passive player, to a scenario whereby we guide or steer the athlete's own active learning process via different tools, both verbal and non-verbal.

THE PROCESS OF PRACTICE AND LEARNING...

An understanding of how best to guide the process of acquiring motor skills is typically something practitioners develop independently with time and experience. Certainly the theory and practice of coaching is often not extensively taught in any meaningful way – if at all, depending on the discipline concerned. Clearly this is a major omission given that these factors will affect how well the athlete not only acquires movement skills in the first instance, but also how we manage the process of refining and re-learning skills over time.

Many practitioners will have heard mention of such terms as implicit learning, external versus internal cues, constraints-based coaching, and even dynamical systems theory. However, these concepts are shrouded in mystery (arguably that is the intention for some who claim expertise in the area) and are often incompletely understood. In this chapter we will attempt to demystify these areas, offering an overview of the basic tenets of these concepts, and explaining the terms employed using plain language.

More importantly we can put these ideas into context to give clarity on why these considerations might be important in the learning process (i.e. why should you care). In turn, we will explore how we might practically account for these aspects when coaching an athlete.

LEARNING AS PROBLEM SOLVING...

So let's begin with a (re)definition of the process by which movement skills are acquired. In essence, learning and ultimately mastering new movements can viewed as a (guided) search for movement solutions for the particular task.

"Practice... (is) a form of exploratory behaviour, a continually evolving search for task solutions"

— Karl M. Newell and Paul V. McDonald (1992) [2]

An important starting point is for the athlete to have a clear understanding of the task - i.e. what the parameters of the task are, and what objective they are aiming to achieve. When coaching a movement we must first define the task, including what constitutes a successful outcome. The athlete needs to know the rules of the game, so should also be equipped with a complete understanding of the constraints involved. In turn this information must also be communicated to the athlete in a way that is comprehensible and meaningful.

Practically, communicating this information may involve demonstrating the movement, or in this Information Age perhaps employing visual media such as video showing another athlete performing the movement task successfully and with a degree of mastery. These themes were covered in the preceding chapter.

Once the athlete is clear on the nature of the task, the next step in the learning process will be exploring what options or solutions are available to them in order to achieve the desired task outcome.

DEFINING PARAMETERS...

Performing a movement task by definition involves the athlete interacting with their environment in order to achieve a defined outcome. The nature of the task and the environment in which the athlete is performing the task impose certain constraints.

Some parameters of the environment are constant and apply equally to all individuals. For instance, gravity and Newtonian laws of motion apply whoever you are. In ecological psychology parlance these consistent 'laws' that are common to all task environments as termed 'invariants'.

Within the aforementioned inviolable invariant constraints (notably the laws of physics), exploring the task environment allows the individual to establish what interactions are possible. The range of interactions that are available to the athlete are framed in the context of their own bodily constraints and capabilities. Exploring within these boundaries allows the athlete to come up with potential movement solutions.

As mentioned, the range of options or 'playbook of movement solutions' available to the athlete will differ according to not only their specific bodily constraints (e.g. height, limb length), but also their capacities (e.g. strength qualities) and capabilities (mobility, global 'athleticism' etc). To some extent this will be dynamic. The athletes' capacities and capabilities can be developed over time; in turn this will alter the potential movement solutions that are available to them.

The constraints associated with both the athlete themselves and the environment in which they must operate will therefore together serve to define the parameters of the movement puzzle and the potential solutions that are available to them.

EXPLORING MOVEMENT OPTIONS...

It is important to understand that the way the athlete perceives the task environment or movement landscape is scaled to their own body and their own perceived capabilities. This is known as 'embodied cognition' of the task environment [3].

As a result of this embodied cognition, the task and the environment in which the task is performed are interpreted by the athlete according to what they afford, in terms of opportunities for action. In other words, the athlete perceives the possibilities for negotiating the task and how they might interact with the task environment relative to their own bodily constraints and capabilities. This defines what the athlete perceives to be the options or movement strategies that are available to them.

Directly perceiving the environment in which we operate allows us to evaluate 'affordances for action'. Affordances therefore represent the opportunities that we perceive to be available to us, with respect to the different ways we can interact with the task environment to achieve an outcome. In this way we can directly perceive the different options and movement strategies we deem to be available to meet our objective.

PERCEIVING AFFORDANCES FOR ACTION...

The concepts of embodied cognition, 'direct perception', and affordances for action, allow us to understand the exploratory process by which we come up with and test out different solutions to a given movement task. These frameworks also explain how the movement solutions that emerge differs between individuals, according to their respective capabilities and problem-solving processes.

The ability to perceive affordances also represents a skill. Part of what constitutes athleticism is possessing highly developed body awareness and a sense of one's own action capabilities. An athlete's level of somatic or bodily awareness can be developed over time. In turn, this will allow us to better perceive our task environment.

By extension, our sense of 'action-scaled affordances', for instance the limits of how high I can reach when I jump, are also developed over time, via related experiences [4]. These affordances or opportunities for action are also dynamic. For instance, with training our capacities and capabilities can be improved. There is therefore a need to continually recalibrate our perception to the shifting limits of our capacities and capabilities [5].

ADAPTIVE LEARNING...

One of the most important things to understand with the process of practice and motor learning is that the athlete's movement behaviour or problem-solving is *adaptive*. This is a process that evolves over time. For instance, as the athlete trials different movement strategies they will discard what worked less well. Ultimately they will settle on, and continue to refine, the select few movement solutions that proved most successful. In ecological dynamics terms this is known as 'emergent behaviour' [6].

> "Practice (is) not repeating the solution of a motor problem time after time, but the process of solving this problem again and again by techniques changed and perfected from repetition to repetition"
>
> — N.A. Bernstein [7]

In addition to direct perception, the trial and error process of experimenting with different solutions is underpinned by the cognitive processes that take place between trials. These internal processes of evaluating previous attempts, reflecting on it, and then planning changes and refinements for subsequent efforts can be complemented with appropriate feedback.

As such, what occurs during the intervals between attempts is integral to the learning process. The provision of feedback should not be excessive during these intervals. We want to avoid constraining the athlete's own problem-solving process. Excessive 'extrinsic' feedback from a coach following attempts can also inhibit the athlete from attending to the feedback that is intrinsic to the action of performing the task. This information is directly available to them without our intervention, so we should not distract them from it.

Aside from refining movement strategies, the process of experimenting and trialling a variety of movement solutions in itself has value. This exploration allows the athlete to build up a movement playbook or repertoire of workable solutions. In turn this provides the 'redundancy' and 'adaptive variability' that are the hallmarks of expert performance [6]. In other words, the athlete is equipped with plan B and plan C options to call upon if circumstances call for it.

ALLOWING FREEDOM TO EXPLORE...

So what is the role of the practitioner in all this? At first glance it seems logical to expedite the process by telling the athlete what the solution is and coaching them through it in great detail. In broad terms this would be characterised as 'explicit learning'.

Unfortunately, whilst this might appear to save time, allowing the athlete some freedom to work through the movement task with a degree of autonomy to come up with the solution(s) themselves may lead to more robust and adaptable learning.

As we have spoken about, providing too much explicit information during practice can impede the athlete from attending to intrinsic feedback and salient information that is directly available to them. Likewise, being too directive in our coaching might inhibit the process of exploring different solutions, and thereby constrain the range and variety of movement solutions that emerge.

Proponents of implicit learning also argue that autonomous learning results in motor skills that are less susceptible to breaking down under pressure. It is argued that 'over-coaching' and providing too much explicit instruction during the learning process may set the athlete up to fail or 'choke' when they ultimately come to perform the task under pressure such as in competition. The rationale is that providing explicit knowledge of the minutiae of the mechanics of the movement when learning can predispose the individual to reverting back and attempting to consciously control skill execution at a later stage, when it should be a well-learned and relatively automated action.

These debates aside, it does follow that movement skills acquired, refined and mastered via exploration and discovery are likely to be more adaptable.

Even for 'closed skill' (predetermined, self-paced) tasks, changes in environmental conditions will clearly alter the constraints of the task, albeit perhaps only subtly. For more complex 'open skill' sports the movement puzzle to be solved and associated constraints involved are constantly changing.

Finally, in the case of high-speed movements and ballistic actions (jumping, sprinting etc) there is similarly a need to avoid 'overthinking', and to minimise cognitive 'noise' that can interfere with and disrupt rapid movement execution. Once again, this would suggest that explicit instruction should be used sparingly, particularly once the athlete has mastered the fundamentals of the movement.

GUIDING THE DISCOVERY PROCESS...

So, does this make coaching redundant? Should the practitioner just sit back and let the athlete work it out for themselves, without any guidance or feedback? Well, no. Even 'exploratory' or 'discovery-based' learning can benefit from guidance. In this way we can avoid having to work through the innumerable possible 'wrong' movement solutions before finally arriving at what works.

Moreover the notion that the athlete will spontaneously self-organise and come up with optimal movement strategies is somewhat questionable.

From an ecological dynamics perspective, coaching might therefore be conceptualised as guiding the athlete's exploration of the practice workspace [8]. Being pragmatic, 'explicit' instruction should be provided sparingly and deliberately during the learning process, rather than not at all. We should of course be mindful of the potential negative consequences of excessive or inappropriate explicit instruction and extrinsic feedback. This does not mean that we abandon these coaching tools entirely.

There are also various tools or 'tricks' that allow coaching information to be provided without direct explicit instruction and extrinsic feedback. For instance, even if explicit instruction is withheld entirely, it is possible to 'channel' the learning process and steer the athlete towards more optimal movement solutions via different methods.

One of the most simple means of steering motor learning in an indirect way involves the use of questioning. This method allows us to assist the athlete in the process of working out the movement puzzle. Well-chosen questions can direct the athlete's attention to salient information within the practice environment. In this way we can similarly direct the athlete to relevant aspects of the task, or elements that are critical to a successful outcome. Essentially we can shine a torch, assisting the athlete's own problem-solving, and guiding them towards more optimal movement solutions.

MANIPULATING THE TASK ENVIRONMENT...

Another 'indirect' approach that stimulates and steers implicit learning is by manipulating constraints in the 'perceptual-motor workspace' during practice. This approach is termed 'constraints-based coaching'. When implemented correctly this can serve to steer the athlete away from common movement errors, and towards more desirable movement behaviours or solutions.

Practically, this may involve the use of actual physical constraints or obstacles during practice. For example, running over low hurdles can prompt the athlete to spontaneously adopt favourable mechanics for sprinting.

Alternatively, 'imaginary' rules or 'projected constraints' can be imposed in the practice environment to steer movement behaviour in a similar fashion [9]. For instance, the coach might implement additional conditions that must be satisfied during practice trials. These constraints might outlaw or penalise unwanted behaviours, or steer the athlete towards more desired outcomes.

Alternatively, the 'projected constraints' employed might be in the form of 'instructional metaphors' or other 'augmented information' provided by the coach. In this way the input from the coach can alter how the athlete perceives the task or the context of the practice environment. The more abstract nature of this form of coaching input serves to enrich rather than detracting from the athlete's motor learning process.

THE POWER OF ANALOGY...

The merits of analogy-based coaching have been acknowledged for some time. For these reasons, some consider analogies to be the holy grail when devising coaching cues. Proponents of this approach describe analogy derived learning as a route for quasi implicit learning [10].

The intention with this form of coaching instruction is to plant an idea: the athlete is prompted to visualise the task, the environment, or themselves in a different and more abstract way. The use of analogy to characterise the athletic skill essentially involves a metaphor that represents the mechanics of the movement. An example might be, 'picture your legs as pistons', 'imagine your spine as a chain'.

This approach demands a level of creativity and lateral thinking on the part of the coach. As with any form of cue, a particular metaphor may resonate with a given individual, whereas in other instances the same analogy will not prove effective in communicating the desired information. It is therefore incumbent upon the coach to trial different analogies and come up with alternatives as necessary.

The athlete plays an active role in the process of translating the analogy or metaphor for the task into action. In essence, the athlete paints their own mental picture, which re-frames how they perceive the movement task.

Analogy-based cues may be internally focussed – i.e. on the athlete's own body, as in the previous examples. Alternatively, external cues can be employed that are 'grounded' in the environment and direct the athlete's attention beyond their own body.

Alternatively internal and external cueing can be employed in combination. One such example when coaching sprint acceleration is conceptualising the shin/foot as a pick axe that breaks through the surface of the track to drive a wedge with each step. This is an example of 'grounding' an internal cue in the task environment. Hence the athlete's locus of attention and the action itself is still directed externally to some degree.

TIMING OF FEEDBACK...

In the previous sections we have discussed what to say and how to say it when providing input to steer motor learning. The final consideration in coaching relates to the timing of instruction or feedback provided, or rather when to withhold input.

Judging when to say either nothing at all, or else very little represents an advanced coaching skill that is generally a hallmark of the experienced coach. In order for any autonomous learning to occur clearly the athlete must be afforded the opportunity to try their own solution. Likewise, we should allow them a chance to correct their previous attempt in the first instance before we intervene or offer correction. In this instance the only input might be to ask the athlete what they thought happened, and then perhaps challenge them to fix it with the next attempt.

These considerations become more prevalent as learning advances and the athlete develops a more refined understanding and mastery of the movement challenge. Essentially the practitioner must favour the more experienced or advanced performer with a greater level of autonomy to fix their mistakes.

By extension, allowing the athlete to choose when they receive coaching input or other feedback such as video during practice can be very powerful. Providing the athlete with control of when they receive input and feedback is shown to facilitate skill acquisition, and is associated with other positive outcomes in relation to their experience of practice and perceived competence [11].

INDIVIDUAL SOLUTIONS...

An important conclusion we can draw from our discussions on the process of practice and developing movement solutions is that there is no single universal template for athletic skills.

What we do have are invariant features that apply to all, such as the laws of physics. Clearly any prospective movement solution that violates these laws will not prove successful. Physics will also go some way to determining what permutations for executing an athletic movement are most effective. Within these boundaries there will nevertheless be a bandwidth of effective and successful options.

The particular array or movement playbook for a given task will be specific to the individual. Depending how the athlete is put together and their capabilities there will be a different range of options that are available and appropriate to them. When observing different sports and athletic events it quickly becomes apparent that elite performers demonstrate individual movement signatures, or versions and variations of technical models that are customised to their own physical attributes and capabilities.

THE ATHLETE-COACH DYAD...

Clearly the coach (and practitioner) needs to understand the relevant principles that underpin the skill acquisition process in order to facilitate the athlete's learning. The process of exploring task solutions undoubtedly benefits from guidance; however, what, how and when input is provided are critical factors to ensure we are helping rather than constraining or hindering the adaptive learning process. These concepts and considerations apply in a variety of contexts, beyond initial skill learning, including refining athletic skills, and remodelling and relearning these skills, for instance following injury.

A central theme in all of this is recognising the athlete's role in the process. The athlete must be an active player. As such, the coach or practitioner cannot dictate the process entirely, as this will foster dependency and renders the athlete a passive recipient of instruction.

Equally, we should also not seek to negate any cognitive involvement on the part of the athlete. Whilst these ideas have some merit, we should not embrace implicit learning to the extent that it is our objective that the athlete is entirely unaware during the learning process and so never develops any level of understanding or expertise.

As will become a theme in these chapters, there is a third way. We can allow freedom for the athlete to explore different movement solutions whilst still helping to guide the process, and highlighting salient information to assist the athlete's learning in relation to the task. Over time, the athlete will assume an increasingly active role in the process.

As the athlete acquires deeper understanding and greater expertise we should enlist them more and more in helping to guide practice. Clearly the athlete's perception is highly pertinent to the process, so it is important to capture this information. We should also allow for the possibility that over time the athlete may become so finely attuned to the skill that what they perceive is actually more accurate than the coach's observation [12]. Similarly, in recognition of this growing awareness and expertise we should allow greater opportunity for the athlete to input into planning and programming, so that this becomes a shared endeavour.

Section Two – Learning and Developing

The Importance of Being Informed

Whatever the nature of the sport, the coaching structure or system of athlete support, a full 360-degrees of mutual understanding should ultimately be the goal for all parties involved (athlete, coach, practitioners). Achieving this mutual understanding requires a level of shared knowledge of the essentials, which in turn necessitates each player in the process becoming better informed not only within their own area, but also across the other respective domains. The ability to converse in a common language will pose unique challenges according to the member of the team concerned. In this chapter we will consider the perspectives of each respective player within the athlete's support team. By definition this will necessarily involve considering the role of the athlete themselves.

INFORMED ATHLETE...

Beginning with the athlete, there is clearly a need for a level of understanding of the technicalities of their sport and their role from a tactical and competition context. This implies a need to acquire a level of technical and tactical knowledge.

Champion athletes tend to be scholars of their sport or event. At the very least the athlete needs to have a clear understanding of what the coach requires of them and the rationale behind it.

Having an understanding of the 'why' as well as what the coach is trying to achieve is very powerful. This a key factor in determining what level of traction the message or coaching intervention ultimately has with the athlete.

From the athlete's viewpoint it is equally important to gain a level of understanding of each aspect of their physical performance and the factors which support it. The success of any interaction or intervention is predicated upon the athlete having a clear idea of the purpose and intention that lies behind it.

Once more this implies a need for the athlete to be informed on the fundamentals of the particular area of sports science, sports medicine, therapy, nutrition etc. This is the only way to ensure the support they receive in the respective area is most effective.

INFORMED PRACTITIONER...

We will turn our attention now to practitioners and associated support staff. Ultimately the knowledge they possess in their respective field of expertise is only as meaningful as their ability to communicate the essential information to the coaches and athletes they support.

The onus is on the practitioner to make the case for the support they offer. Ultimately the practitioner needs to take the time to understand the needs of the athlete and coach. It is futile presenting them with a solution until we have taken the time to understand what problems they actually want to solve.

More specifically, for the coach and athlete to buy in, clearly they need to know how the service on offer is ultimately going to make them better able to prepare and compete in their sport. Equally it is important to not oversell the benefits. We are not trying to justify our existence but rather add value and act in service to the coach and athlete.

"Let the main thing stay the main thing"

— Brendan Venter MD

The practitioner must also be sufficiently self-aware to recognise their own work in the context of the overall priorities of the athlete, the coach, and the situation at hand. This demands not only humility but empathy.

There is an argument that if the practitioner or member of support staff lacks the emotional intelligence to be a 'coach' they have no business interacting directly with the athlete. At the very least, practitioners must respect the role of the coach as 'gatekeeper', and be willing to follow agreed protocol for communicating feedback. In essence, the practitioner should be prepared to invest the time to acquire the status of a coach in order to earn the right to have a direct line of communication with the athlete.

In the same way, in order to operate effectively and for the coach and athlete support structure to function properly, each member of staff must understand the context of the realms in which they operate. Effective athlete support necessitates a breadth and depth of knowledge of the sport, the support team, and the environment in which the athletes and coaches operate. Ultimately everything should be geared to supporting the coach and the athlete.

From this viewpoint, understanding the necessary details becomes essential. If the practitioner does not take the time to understand the performance model and specific objectives the coach and athlete are working towards they cannot have a true appreciation of how they might add value in supporting the coach and athlete in working towards these outcomes.

INFORMED COACH...

Moving on finally to the coach, as the leader and director of the programme the coach must possess the greatest array of knowledge spanning across a number of different areas.

"Do coaches need to be therapists, nutritionists or biomechanists? No. But they should have a good understanding to be able to communicate with their network of people"

— Dan Pfaff

When operating in a multidisciplinary team a key role of the coach is that of gate keeper. However, to fulfil this role effectively requires a breadth of knowledge across each domain. Clearly, it is very difficult to steer support and make informed decisions on what input the athlete is exposed to when if you only have a vague idea of what each practitioner involved actually does.

Another aspect where this understanding across domains is critical is in order for the coach to be able to select the best staff to provide this support for their athletes. In the interests of quality control, their knowledge must be sufficient that they are able to distinguish good practice versus poor practice.

A key element of being a leader and having the propensity to direct athlete support involves possessing the requisite knowledge to be able to interrogate the each member of the support team on their respective area of support. Clearly an understanding of the terms involved is helpful in this way, so that coach and practitioner are speaking the same language. However, beyond this the coach must possess a depth of knowledge in order to engage in informed debate.

A FINAL THOUGHT…

It can be said that a good coach is a curious coach. Indeed, an innate desire to discover is a common trait shared by good coaches, practitioners, and athletes. For practitioners in particular a willingness to step outside their domain to observe and adopt the role of learner. This requires bravery and is a test of the ability to put their ego and status to one side. The willingness of those involved to take these steps and engage in the learning process will reveal much about what motivates their practice. Those who are truly committed to serving the athlete should prove receptive to these initiatives, regardless of how discomfiting they find the prospect.

Challenges in the Quest for Continuing Education and Professional Development

Practitioners' motivation for undertaking continuing professional development (CPD) and continuing education activities varies. Inevitably part of this pursuit is to fulfil the ongoing requirements of professional accreditation and certifications. Equally, for the majority there is also a genuine wish to improve practice and, perhaps to a lesser extent, their knowledge and understanding of various topics (more on that later).

PROFESSIONAL DEVELOPMENT OPPORTUNITIES ARE NOT CREATED EQUAL...

For those seeking to develop their skills and knowledge the process of selecting which resources to buy and what courses and workshops to attend can be a challenge. In many instances CPD courses, workshops, online quizzes and even books are 'endorsed' to earn credits with respective certifying bodies or professional organisations (ACSM, NATA, NSCA to name a few). Whilst this accreditation process offers some reassurance on the content delivered, in reality in many instances this process is largely about the provider paying the fee.

Moreover many professional and regulatory bodies make little distinction between CPD activities so that all are essentially treated as equal. In this case there is no real quality control from 'above', so that the onus once more rests with the individual practitioner to assess the rigour and merit of the many CPD courses, seminars, and workshops on offer.

THE CHALLENGE OF CONTINUING EDUCATION...

Continuing education is another area where practitioners face challenges. Often when a practitioner's enrolment in tertiary education ends so does the free access to academic journals that comes with it. This is clearly unfortunate. The period following qualification when they are first starting to practice is arguably the time when practitioners most need access to these resources.

There are some very good online information sources that the practitioner can use to stay up to date with what research literature that is coming out. If used wisely, social media channels such as twitter can be helpful here.

Nevertheless road blocks will often still arise when attempting to access the full content. The costs of subscribing to multiple journals are prohibitive. Some prominent journals are offering more open access content, however the cost of buying or renting single publications that are not free to access is often quite ridiculous.

So what is the solution? For those with the time to search there are a variety of sources of information that are available online and free to access.

PERILS OF THE VIRTUAL WORLD...

When exploring online and various sources including social media there is such a massive volume of content available that the challenge becomes one of filtering.

Much of the information that is freely available online is also incomplete. Clearly much of the value (and certainly all of the nuance) is lost when the source we are working from is the abstract of a research paper, or some other summary, such as the ubiquitous infographic.

A great deal of caution is required when exploring the virtual realm. Without the peer-review process, or any requirement for the author to declare competing interests, once more it comes down to the individual to make a subjective value judgement on both the content and the source.

Clearly this can be something of a minefield, particularly for less experienced practitioners and those who lack extensive knowledge in the particular area. There are a host of online experts posting their philosophy and funky looking training videos via various online and social media channels.

THE RISE OF THE VIRTUAL EXPERT...

We are approaching a tipping point whereby online profile is becoming accepted as a proxy for professional standing. Arguably online profile and social media presence are becoming valued on a par with actual experience and demonstrated expertise. The validation offered by an online audience is fast replacing professional reputation that is earned on merit.

The rise of the virtual expert is a worrisome trend, and I fear one that will only continue to grow. Often those who claim online guru status embellish or even invent their professional experience, and claim associations that are either spurious or outright untrue. In doing so they take advantage of the protection offered by the remote nature of the virtual medium, and the fact that all too frequently they are not called on their duplicity.

It follows that the most inexperienced are most prone to the influence of online gurus. That said, even established practitioners and authorities in the field are falling into the trap of associating with dubious characters on the strength of their online profile and the size of their following. Unwittingly in doing so they lend their credibility to these virtual experts, which of course only strengthens their standing.

PRACTICAL WORKSHOPS...

For a variety of reasons the energy and financial costs involved with pursuing continuing education can become too much, and many would rather invest their time and money in something they can use in their practice. Most often this involves attending workshops and courses offering the opportunity to learn practical techniques and information that can be taken away and directly applied to practice.

Yet here too healthy scepticism can be an important ally. The sad reality is that many of these events are run with the purpose of promoting a brand and selling product. There are numerous examples of the tail of commercial interests wagging the dog of professional practice.

The truth is that practice in the field is heavily influenced by marketing and promotion, arguably more so than empirical evidence. Most practitioners can readily call to mind products and practices that were popularised in this way, and later found to have little or no scientific merit.

TO SUM UP...

Evidence-led practice requires that practitioners invest the time and embrace the challenges we will inevitably encounter on the path to becoming better informed. It seems appropriate that this should be an obligation that practitioners must fulfil in order to maintain their professional certification.

The message for those embarking on this journey is essentially: go forth, but do so armed with a filter and healthy dose of scepticism to hand. We will dig deeper into the need to embrace scepticism and guard our faculties for critical thinking in a later chapter.

Ego is the Enemy of Progress and Discovery

It is a commonly held view that ego stunts personal growth, and most would agree that ego undermines our effectiveness as coaches and practitioners. What is less often considered is that unconstrained ego similarly obstructs progress and discovery in the areas of scientific study that exist to inform practice. At present the respective disciplines encompassed within coaching science, sports science and sports medicine are plagued with these difficulties. Einstein famously quoted to the effect that ego has an inverse relationship to knowledge – "more the knowledge, lesser the ego; lesser the knowledge, more the ego". Yet researchers in the fields of sports science and sports medicine are showing themselves to be particularly prone to ego and the excesses associated with it. In this chapter we tackle the issue of ego in sports science and sport medicine, and attempt to plot a path back to sanity.

THE PRESENT SITUATION...

Observing the conduct and interactions between prominent researchers and 'authorities' in the fields of sports science and sports medicine can make for an unedifying spectacle. In the era of social media these petulant and very public spats are becoming increasingly common. These displays do no credit to anybody involved. Worse, these developments actively obstruct rational discussion that might actually help to solve the problem we set out to resolve in the first place.

This trend has recently prompted calls for reason that cite the increasingly extreme positions taken by prominent researchers and 'authorities' [13]. The increasing 'extremism' also extends into how debates on particular topics are conducted. In his writing Ross Tucker has used the analogy of a pendulum to describe the present situation. Periodically the pendulum swings from one extreme viewpoint on a topic to the opposite extreme. Clearly the present situation serves nobody.

In particular, for students and practitioners who are seeking to become better informed the present situation makes for baffling viewing, and is entirely unhelpful from a learning viewpoint. Hereby those of us who are involved in sports science and medicine research are actively failing those we are meant to serve.

ASK A GROWN UP...

Of all the sciences, what we consider sports science is one of the youngest and least evolved. It therefore makes sense to take our lead from more established areas of scientific study. In essence, let's examine what the grown-ups do.

Here we turn to physics, one the longest established of the sciences. Physics is not only eminently relevant to what we do, but also gives us some valuable principles to follow. Throughout this chapter we will call upon the wisdom of Richard Feynman as our guide.

ALL IS UNCERTAIN...

The more we understand about the universe it becomes increasingly clear that uncertainty is an inherent feature.

"Scientific knowledge is a body of statements of varying degrees of certainty... some most unsure, some nearly sure, none absolutely certain..."

– Richard Feynman

In essence, our understanding of everything is at best clouded and incomplete. What we 'know' is merely our current best guess or approximation based on the evidence presently available. Knowledge is inconstant and fleeting. This is a critical realisation. It should also serve as an important lesson in humility. Moreover this understanding should give us pause about becoming too attached to what we 'know' to be 'true'.

"To make progress in understanding, we must remain modest and allow that we do not know"

– Richard Feynman

DOUBT AND FALLIBILITY...

"This permanent doubt, the deep source of science..."

– Carlo Rovelli [14]

Doubt is at the very core of science. It is also entirely appropriate given the uncertainty that is inherent in scientific study and our tenuous grip on knowledge. We should be reassured by the fact that even the great minds in history who were responsible for the major advances in science and our understanding of the universe showed suitable hesitancy and doubt as they proposed their great discoveries [14].

"A scientist is never certain... We absolutely must leave room for doubt, or there is no progress and there is no learning"

– Richard Feynman

By extension, denying that we are ourselves fallible is not only unhelpful but is also ridiculous. Fallibility is an inevitable part of being a human engaging in scientific study. Fallibility is a necessary and integral part of the process of discovery. Einstein is rightly heralded for his extraordinary scientific genius. Yet we overlook that Einstein repeatedly (and publicly) proposed solutions that were wrong on his way to arriving at his great discoveries.

SCIENTIFIC PROCESS (SEE CRIMES AGAINST)...

The basis of accepted scientific method as established by Karl Popper is falsifiability. Accordingly, hypothesis testing should essentially be a quest to disprove the initial proposition through experiment. This is a process of natural selection. The very objective of scientific study is to stress test and actively try to disprove the hypothesis. In the end it is the hypotheses that withstand this rigorous process that survive.

Once a body of evidence in support of the hypothesis has been amassed via experimentation, the hypothesis attains the status of a theory. Hence what defines and differentiates a theory is that there is empirical evidence to support it from a number of experimental studies.

There are two critical points here. The first is that by definition it is impossible to propose a theory – at the outset it is merely an untested hypothesis. Increasingly the two terms are used interchangeably in the literature, and this is a real problem as it erodes the standards of proof.

The second point is that even when a proposition attains the status of 'theory' following an extended period of scientific study it is never considered proven beyond doubt. Critical thinking and scientific enquiry should be applied with an established theory just as with a hypothesis.

THE REALITY OF SPORTS SCIENCE RESEARCH...

We should acknowledge here that in reality there are a variety of agendas at play which drive research output and influence the selection of topics for scientific investigation in sports science and sports medicine. Advancing knowledge or striving for scientific discovery for its own sake tend to be lost amidst these more pressing concerns for career academics.

In the dog eat dog world of academia, young researchers (and those who are not so young) are often seeking the latest hot topic that will make their name. Consequently, most often researchers have a vested interest in the success of the research proposal. In this way the proposition becomes inextricably linked with the researcher's own advancement. In turn, promoting the idea becomes a vehicle for promoting themselves, particularly in the social media era.

Clearly these agendas have nothing to do with scientific discovery. Indeed they are in fact contrary to it. Such agendas foster an unhealthy attachment to our proposition, and this inevitably impacts how we behave towards others in the field.

Against this backdrop, from the outset of the life of a hypothesis scientific method too often soon deviates from the accepted process of critical enquiry. Instead of actually testing the hypothesis (i.e. trying to disprove it), there is a strong motivation to rather seek to generate evidence to support it. So eager are we to find support that the temptation is to rig the conditions of the experiment to give ourselves every chance of a positive finding. Clearly this is a violation of the whole premise of critical enquiry and scientific process.

AUTHORITIES AND 'DISSENT'...

Unhealthy attachment to a hypothetical model or view of the world is one of the biggest barriers to discovery and learning. As we have spoken about, the level of attachment is likely to be all the more strong if we feel ownership of the idea. When it is 'our idea', or our stated position, this becomes entangled with our ego. As such, we are more likely to take challenges personally. This also raises the stakes, as there are consequences if we are deemed to be 'wrong'.

Indeed we become so attached to our best guesses or proposed solutions that too often we abandon any commitment to actually exploring the question. In the face of challenge, we fall into an adversarial mode of staunchly defending our position and our proposition, rather than scrutinising our own preconceived ideas and entertaining alternative viewpoints.

In the present climate too often we are seeing prominent researchers and territorial research groups who aggressively seek to shut down dissent and attack those who have the temerity to disagree or to question.

Clearly such a situation is not only toxic, but it is also insupportable. There is no monopoly on knowledge. Nobody should be considered, or consider themselves, above having their findings or propositions questioned.

"There is no authority who decides what is a good idea"

– Richard Feynman

As we have spoken about, a key tenet of science is that nothing is ever proven. Hypotheses and theories must remain subject to questioning and critical scientific investigation. Even once the basic premise has been stress tested via experimentation, we should continue to actively explore and establish conditions and populations for which the proposition does not hold true.

FALSE PROPHETS...

Given the uncertainty and precarious nature of scientific 'knowledge', it is startling the over-confidence and absolute certainty that is projected by proponents of a particular school of thought on topics in sports science and sports medicine.

We increasingly find prominent figures and research groups presenting themselves as an authority, or worse still the sole rightful authority on a particular area of study. In the most extreme cases, individuals are claiming ownership of an aspect of training, a type of injury, or even a whole body part or muscle group ('The Glute Guy').

Sadly we must accept some responsibility for this, as we are somewhat complicit. A false prophet is nothing without followers. We want to believe. So unnerved are we by the notion of uncertainty that we embrace self-proclaimed authorities for the artificial and quite false sense of certainty this gives us. We are comforted by the illusion that somebody knows and has the answers.

"The scientific spirit distrusts whoever claims to be the one having ultimate answers, or privileged access to Truth"

– Carlo Rovelli [14]

A revelation: nobody has it all figured out. Those who project such a ridiculous notion of themselves are either deluded or ignorant (perhaps both).

There is of course still room for pioneers. However the real value of pioneers has always been that they see the world differently. Bringing a different perspective or viewing the same problem in a different way opens up a host of new potential solutions to others. The crucial point is that nobody has ownership over an idea or field of scientific enquiry.

NO PROGRESS WITHOUT QUESTIONING…

Through a combination of realism and humility, we should be ever conscious of the limits of our collective knowledge on any given topic. Accordingly, we should also leave room to doubt the veracity of what is currently 'known'. There is no such thing as a definitive answer in science; we should continue to examine the problem and scrutinise the solutions that have been proposed.

Deference should have no place in science. Absolutely we should respect what has gone before; however, this does not mean these established ideas are sacrosanct and above scrutiny. Advances in science and knowledge only become possible when we cast aside the blind faith that our elders and betters know best. A prerequisite for progress is finding the courage to re-examine the problem, regardless of whether it is considered 'solved', and entertain the possibility of alternative solutions.

One of the biggest obstacles in the present climate particularly is the default response to alternative viewpoints, and 'challengers' who present different ideas on a topic.

When our ideas are challenged we are too quick to take offence, and assume there is some slight intended. Likewise we see an alternative viewpoint that challenges the dominant school of thought we automatically assume some attempt to dethrone the incumbent. This is essentially killing scientific debate, particularly in public forums, such as social media. We need to change how we entertain challenge, and our attitude to disagreement.

Another revelation: it is possible to have differing perspectives; this does not discredit what has gone before. Different points of view can co-exist. There is no insult in questioning existing ideas or proposing alternative solutions. The act of disagreeing, or rather not completely agreeing, does not imply any disrespect.

We need to find a way to separate our ego from what should be the shared quest for discovery. The elements of questioning, exploring different perspectives, and respectful disagreement are the life blood of scientific discovery and progress. To that end we should embrace such challenges and enthusiastically engage in debate; these are the very things that stimulate new ideas and innovations.

BACK TO REALITY...

Sports science is one of the youngest and least evolved of all the sciences. Moreover, it is also one of the least exact. A feature of biological systems is inherent variability, including variation both between and within populations. There are no absolutes. When dealing with sentient humans particularly, there are also a host of confounding factors.

Everything is inexact. Always it is dependent on context. What we see will depend on the population involved, and further on where the individual sits on the spectrum within that population.

Let us return to a fundamental point that we opened the chapter with: sports science and sports medicine exist to inform practice. This critical realisation has become lost on many within academic circles. If the way in which research is conducted is at odds with valid scientific enquiry, or the behaviour of the individuals involved does not serve this higher aim, those responsible should be called out and held to account for their offences.

Returning to Einstein's notion that ego has an inverse relationship with knowledge, if we have acquired knowledge, but are not able to separate our ego from this knowledge, then we are ultimately ignorant.

From the learners' viewpoint, we should not unquestioningly accept anything that is written or presented to us. Equally neither should we refuse to entertain others' positions and dismiss them out of hand. There is a third way, as we explore in the following chapter.

Resurrecting Critical Thinking

I n the Information Age the propensity for critical thinking has become arguably the most critical skill. With unprecedented access to a vast sea of information at the touch of a key stroke, the ability to filter and to critically evaluate are paramount. This is the great irony of the Information Age; at a time when the need has never been greater, critical thinking is seemingly a dying art. Increasingly we are plagued with superficial knowledge and incomplete understanding. We are beset on all sides by spurious reasoning and a preponderance of facile solutions. In this chapter we make the case for resurrecting critical thinking, and attempt to trace a path to rediscovering our faculties for independent learning and freedom of thought.

GROUP THINK AND THE TEMPTATIONS OF A GOOD STORY...

In 2017 I wrote a guest article entitled 'Crimes Against Critical Thinking in the Face of a Good Story'. This was something of a call to arms for enemies of 'group think' and defenders of critical thinking.

"Whenever you find yourself on the side of the majority, it is time to pause and reflect"

— Mark Twain

More specifically, the theme of the article related to the manner in which popularised concepts or practices, and the hype that surrounds them, is received by practitioners in different domains. In the article I described an often observed phenomenon, which can be summed up by the phrase 'never let the truth get in the way of a good story'. Essentially, if the narrative presented appeals to a particular bias or something we wish to be true, we tend to unwittingly, yet quite willingly, suspend our critical thinking.

It is beguilingly easy to succumb to own cognitive bias in the face of a message we find appealing. We must recognise and reconcile ourselves to the fact that we are prone to bias and prejudice. We must acknowledge our biases, and how they can affect our reasoning, in order to resist.

FLAWS IN THE EDUCATION PROCESS...

"Education is not the learning of facts, but the training of the mind to think"

— Albert Einstein

In the excellent article by Prof Daniel T Willingham [15], he delves into difficulties of fostering critical thinking in modern education. Whilst most in education would agree on the need to provide these skills to the learner, as Willingham writes there is no real consensus on what specifically critical thinking comprises.

Certainly, what attempts have been made to teach these higher order skills have to date been largely unsuccessful. A possible reason for this is that critical thinking represents a way of viewing the world, entertaining and assimilating new information, and engaging in independent thought and reasoning. There are parallels here with fostering abstract abilities such as creativity and problem-solving.

SOURCING INFORMATION...

There are an increasing number of instances where social media is becoming the predominant source of information for the practitioner. Social media is often a great way to be alerted to new research or topical ideas and practices in the field. However, it remains critical to then seek out the source to discover more.

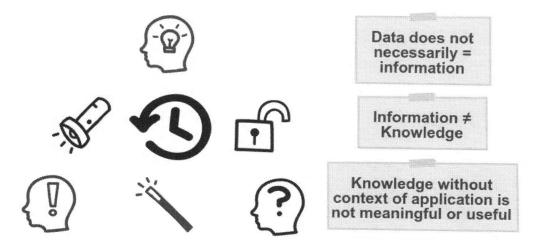

Figure 1: Data, Information, Knowledge, Understanding

Too often practitioners are relying on soundbites or a snapshot, without taking the time to read the full content and independently evaluate the data presented. Essentially if the full extent of your information comes from an abstract or an infographic, you have fallen at the first hurdle.

By definition, the critical thinking process is contingent on first having the full information at your disposal. Sadly, getting access to this information often presents a challenge and can prove costly without open source publishing, or resources that provide a synthesis of current literature.

That said, in this new era of connectivity it is often possible to reach out to the source. My experience is that authors, practitioners and coaches are often amenable to having a conversation and responding to questions.

GATHERING INTELLIGENCE AND SCRUTINIZING INFORMATION...

Sourcing (and then reading) the relevant information and literature available should be viewed as intelligence gathering. With the seas of information available, our ability to filter becomes a critical skill.

The process of intelligence gathering can be greatly expedited if our search can be directed to the most complete sources of information, and bypass what is not useful. That said, whilst there is very little we should swallow whole, there is usually something we can take from most publications or information sources.

It is equally critical to consider what you are using this information for. If you use what you have read as a shield to defend a position, this should be a warning sign. Likewise, if you find yourself simply parroting what you have read, this should also give you pause.

We must be clear in our aim, which ultimately is to derive an independent and balanced conclusion on the topic that considers a variety of sources and diverging perspectives.

AN OPEN MIND ALLIED WITH HEALTHY SCEPTICISM...

Returning to the notion of intelligence gathering, clearly we must retain an open mind in order to entertain new ideas, even if they differ to what we presently believe to be true.

"Scepticism is the process of applying reason and critical thinking to determine validity. It's the process of finding a supported conclusion, not the justification of a preconceived conclusion."

— Brian Dunning

Another part of the intelligence gathering process is that we must consider the source. We must consider their motivation (and possible agendas), in relation to how the information is presented and the message that is conveyed. We must independently evaluate the data, and weigh the evidence, in order to establish whether the data in fact support the conclusions presented. We then take what makes sense and add it as a piece in the jigsaw.

ACKNOWLEDGING OUR OWN BIAS AND PREJUDICE...

As noted in the second part of the quote above, just as we must evaluate the source and the motivations of the authors, we must also consider our own preconceptions.

As we spoke about earlier, the process and level of scrutiny applied should be the same whether or not the view presented aligns with our opinion or bias. We cannot become lax or suspend our critical thinking simply because we find the message agreeable. We must scrutinise every assumption.

An important realisation for any practitioner is that we are as prone to systematic error due to our own bias as anybody. We cannot underestimate the degree to which we are prone to misjudgement.

A crucial starting point therefore is to accept our fallibility. With this acceptance we can start to become aware of our own particular cognitive biases. Armed with this awareness, we can then take appropriate steps and employ countermeasures to resist the different sources of bias we are likely to encounter.

Periodically we should also critically evaluate our opinions on various topics and the assumptions that underpin them. Nothing should be beyond scrutiny.

IN CLOSING...

In our quest to resurrect critical thinking we have explored some of the challenges and pitfalls faced by practitioners and coaches in this era of connectivity, mobile technology and social media. We have also described the key steps in the process of critical thinking. Our task begins with 'intelligence gathering', whereby we source and filter the information available before independently evaluating the data presented.

As we have discussed we must retain both an open mind to entertain new concepts and ideas, and also healthy scepticism to scrutinise the information and conclusions presented. We must also apply the same scrutiny to our own assumptions and opinions, in order for our understanding to evolve.

Finally, we must synthesise what we have gleaned from a variety of sources to arrive at a balanced and considered view. Each step in the process involves a range of skills; clearly our task is far from straightforward. Nevertheless, for coaches, practitioners, and indeed athletes, critical thinking represents the principal means to remain informed in the Information Age.

Section Three – Mentoring

The Why and How of Mentoring

Mentoring or apprenticeship is a universal path for developing coaches and practitioners across all disciplines. Indeed in many realms mentorship is often the primary means for practical learning, as well as passing on experiential knowledge. Given this, there are surprisingly few resources dedicated to this highly complex and multifaceted process, particularly in the context of performance sport and related vocations. Even the rationale for mentoring seems incomplete. For instance, it is generally assumed what the apprentice or 'mentee' is getting out of the process; however, the motivation and apparent benefit to the person providing the mentoring is not typically considered. In this post we attempt to address this; we will tackle the why as well as the how of mentoring, and explore these aspects from the perspectives of both the mentor and the mentee.

HOW MENTORING SERVES THE MENTOR...

"Teaching is the highest form of understanding"

— Aristotle

According to the pyramid construct of passive and active or participatory forms of learning, teaching (and mentoring) can be considered the highest form of 'participatory' learning. The level of retention with this method of active learning is rated as the highest of all. As such, the process of mentoring represents a means of continuing education for the mentor, just as it is for the one receiving mentoring.

Beyond learning and retention, organising one's thoughts in order to impart acquired knowledge, and the act of delivering this information, are processes that serve to deepen understanding. For instance, in the process of being quizzed by the mentee, the mentor will periodically encounter a question or perspective that they have not considered before. Once again, this exemplifies how both mentor and mentee learn by engaging in the mentoring process.

Moreover, taking on the mantle of 'mentor' in itself encourages one to strive to invest the requisite time and effort to stay up to date. Mentoring inherently provides those concerned with the impetus to continue to broaden their knowledge, so as to remain equipped to deliver learning to those they are mentoring and answer their questions.

THE PROCESS...

The universal starting point when I engage in mentoring involves undertaking a SWOT analysis, whereby the learner evaluates their present strengths and weaknesses in designated areas, and identifies prospective opportunities, as well as potential threats or barriers.

Below are some examples of themes employed to guide the process of identifying signature strengths across relevant areas, as well as present 'weaknesses', or rather areas requiring development:

Theoretical knowledge/understanding	Technical expertise
Programming and prescription	Eye for movement
Instruction techniques	Interaction with athletes

This process provides a starting point for an initial discussion that serves to elucidate priority development areas. Generally, this is limited to two or three items, comprising topical areas of specific interest, and aspects where they identify a particular need to upskill. This process is revisited periodically in order to update and revise the personal development plan on an ongoing basis.

FILLING IN THE BLANKS...

Mentoring essentially bridges the gap between the learner's studies or training in the area and the applied knowledge required to become an effective practitioner in the field. In other words, the task of the mentor is to equip the aspiring practitioner with tools that are not customarily provided in the formal education process, and provide learning in areas not generally well catered for in lectures or textbooks.

Central to the mentoring process is translating 'book learning' and theory into a practical context. Often this involves a realisation that the textbook version of how things work differs to what is evident in practice. The role of the mentor is therefore to provide context and impart to the learner a true appreciation of applied knowledge in practice.

INTERNSHIPS...

Internships have become a mainstay of many professions in elite and professional sport, notably in coaching and physical preparation. As these 'opportunities' are often unpaid, or poorly paid, the main value offered to the intern is in the form of hands-on coaching experience and practical learning, through some combination of mentoring, observation, and the experience of working alongside experienced practitioners with high-level athletes.

Despite the lack of financial compensation, competition for internship placement opportunities is often fierce; this is in part due to the saturation of the marketplace (a notable example is the field of strength and conditioning). Many aspiring practitioners face difficulties getting a foothold in the early part of their journey, and internships are increasingly considered a necessary part of the process of building a career in the 'industry'.

Sadly, the experiences offered to many interns do not meet their needs or expectations. With such a ready supply of free or cheap labour, some organisations abuse the internship process, and simply use interns for menial tasks and provide very little in the way of learning or mentoring in return.

Clearly, all internships were not created equal, so homework is required and it pays to be selective. Equally, if the aspiring practitioner chooses well and is successful in securing a place on reputable internship with people who are invested in the process, the experience can be invaluable and have a significant and lasting impact.

From a personal viewpoint, I regularly take on placement students and provide opportunities for graduates and other practitioners to spend time coaching on a voluntary basis; as part of the arrangement I personally provide individualised professional development and mentoring. I am particularly mindful of my obligations to the placement student or volunteer coach. In the absence of financial compensation it becomes more crucial to fulfil these obligations, by ensuring we provide equal or greater value in relation to time and effort they invest. Indeed I make it clear to the individual that in the event we ever fail to provide the requisite value I fully expect and encourage them to walk away.

THE GIFT OF CURATING INFORMATION SOURCES...

In the Information Age, one of the biggest ways in which a mentor can add value is by directing the practitioner in their search for information. In essence, this the virtue of information curation. Taking advantage of the catalogue of information sources acquired over the period of a career, the mentor can direct their protégé towards quality content on whatever topic they want to learn more about. This simple act can spare a great deal of time spent on fruitless searching, or worse becoming diverted by dubious material.

With the burgeoning resources and information sources available, learning and operating in the Information Age requires a highly developed filter. By definition, this is the very thing that relative novices in the field lack. The ability to discriminate and differentiate quality information from a credible source is a critical skill. The mentor can help direct the search, lend the benefit of their filter, and use the process to school their protégé in critical thinking.

PREPARED...

It is important that novice coaches and practitioners are exposed to interacting with athletes early in the process. That said, throwing them in at the deep end is a high-risk strategy.

Operating in elite sport is not for the faint-hearted; from that viewpoint, an argument can be made that at some point there is a need to see if the individual will sink or swim. Nevertheless, putting a 'green' practitioner into a situation they are not adequately prepared for should be avoided where possible, unless done so intentionally (and with the consent of all parties) to serve a defined purpose or learning outcome.

Failing is to some degree an integral part of the learning process. Equally, putting a relative novice into a situation where they are essentially doomed to failure is basically an act of neglect, and is certainly not conducive to building trust in the relationship moving forward.

FINDING THEIR VOICE...

An essential part of the mentoring process is encouraging the young practitioner to find their own voice, and evolve their own style of coaching. Whilst they might adopt certain traits or behaviours they have observed from others, it is critical that the protégé does not try to copy their mentor or emulate their manner of coaching.

In order to be credible a coach or practitioner must find their own authentic style. Regardless of the discipline or field of practice, the elements of 'coaching' and human interaction are integral to being an effective practitioner in sport. If the individual comes across as false or inauthentic they will fail to earn the respect or trust of the athlete.

AUTONOMY NOT AUTOMATONS...

Returning briefly to the topic of internships, an issue with institute of sport systems in particular is the tendency to seek to indoctrinate and mould interns in their own image. No system or organisation has a monopoly on best practice. It is clearly a fallacy that any one approach is inherently superior. Indeed, seeking to institutionalise in this way is contrary to creating an environment for sustaining best practice and innovation. In that sense, any system that strives to create clones from those entering the organisation is doomed.

Conversely, the traits of inquisitiveness and free thinking should be highly prized and rewarded. As we will delve into in a later chapter, organisations that aspire to be elite should not hire applicants who parrot the most acceptable answers, but rather those who ask the best questions. This message should be emphasised and reinforced throughout the mentoring process.

> "Great leaders do not create more followers; they create more leaders"
>
> — Tom Peters

LETTING GO...

Even for those with a great deal of knowledge to impart, the hardest part of the process often comes in the latter stages of the relationship when the role of the mentee transitions from that of apprentice to becoming more autonomous. From the mentor's viewpoint this requires the ability and readiness to relinquish control when the time comes.

Practically, the preparations for this transition should occur at a much earlier stage in the process, by progressively giving freer rein and greater responsibility to the individual undergoing mentoring.

> "Leaders become great not because of their power but because of their ability to empower others"
>
> — John C. Maxwell

MENTORING EXPERIENCED PRACTITIONERS...

For the most part, so far we have discussed mentoring in relation to practitioners who are in the early stages of their career. However, mentoring is not only for novice practitioners; the benefits of having a mentor are apparent even for coaches and practitioners with many years of experience.

An indicative example is the 'Apprentice Coach Program' provided by Altis, a 'working' track and field training facility that provides education for coaches and practitioners. One notable point about this initiative is the use of the word 'apprentice' in the title, despite the fact that the majority of the coaches and practitioners who attend are highly experienced and well established. This underlines that even experienced and established practitioners recognise the value of apprenticeship (more's the pity it only lasts a week).

Clearly it is critical that the wealth of experience and knowledge that an experienced coach or practitioner brings with them is acknowledged in the mentoring relationship. Most often those who wish to engage in mentoring are seeking to learn from a mentor who has specific expertise in a particular area. In other cases, what the mentor provides is simply an alternative perspective.

The mentoring arrangement with an experienced coach is therefore far more akin to peer learning, as opposed to a hierarchical relationship. The mentoring process in such instances calls for humility on both sides.

> On the topic of ego in coaching: "If you are capable of honesty, and you have spent time in the trenches, sport is humbling every day (and ego isn't an issue)"
>
> — Dan Pfaff

THE FINAL FRONTIER – 'PEER MENTORSHIP'...

Our discussions so far have predominantly considered mentoring in the context of young coaches and practitioners. It is important to note however that there is no stipulation that mentoring needs to be a hierarchical relationship. We should recognise that well established and highly experienced individuals can equally derive a great deal of benefit from a different form of peer-to-peer 'mentoring'.

Simply having somebody to confer with who is external to our normal working environment can bring huge mutual value. Engaging in peer-to-peer discussions can help bring clarity, interactively working through the problem-solving process and shared 'thought experiments' to test the viability of potential solutions. These interactions can also spark ideas for both parties; we will discuss this theme of 'inspiration' in a later chapter.

Sadly, in certain disciplines, notably strength and conditioning, relatively well established practitioners have proven reticent to engage with peers in this way. I would argue that this reticence is most often borne out of fear, insecurity, and the notion that seeking out a colleague for assistance might be perceived as weakness, or harm their standing in some way. That said, recent developments in the field suggest that this mind-set might be shifting somewhat.

We do not necessarily have to employ the terms mentor or mentorship to characterise this peer-to-peer relationship. Labels aside, the important aspect is that we have somebody to provide an objective and informed opinion, and alternative perspectives that we may not have considered. Whether the person providing this service is a more experienced coach or a peer, it is crucial that we have somebody to call upon who is able to challenge our thinking and help to hold ourselves accountable.

Lessons Along the Way – Advice for Young Practitioners

Providing learning opportunities and mentoring to coaches and practitioners has been a recurring theme throughout my career, and I continue to be actively involved in mentoring young coaches and practitioners in the early stages of their career working with athletes. These interactions frequently prompt me to reflect on my own journey and what I have learned on the way. In the absence of a mentor in the early stages of my career I keep circling back to what would have been useful to have been told starting out. This chapter is a collection of twenty-five critical lessons that are pertinent to young practitioners and common to all disciplines.

1. Be informed; knowledge is power.
Expertise is essentially having an appreciation of how much you have yet to learn. Learning is a process without end - and strive for both depth and breadth of knowledge.
2. Ask questions.
Speak up if you don't understand something, you have a query or you require clarification. This isn't about hiding your ignorance; remaining silent gets you nowhere and is an indulgence you cannot afford if you aspire to be elite.
3. Be receptive to being questioned.
Don't view it as a challenge to your authority when somebody asks 'why' in relation to what you prescribe. Rather it is a first step to engaging the athlete (or coach) and getting them on board with what you are trying to do. And if you don't have a good answer then you either need to find one or change your practice.
4. Be clear on the purpose of everything you do.
Superficial understanding won't cut it under interrogation. Drill down to first principles. Have a strong rationale and justification for each element of your programme.
5. Ensure that your athletes are clear on the purpose behind everything in the programme.
Don't assume it is obvious. It may seem like it goes without saying; for your athlete it doesn't necessarily go without saying. Ask the athlete what they think the purpose or rationale of a particular exercise is. If it isn't clear then enlighten them.
6. Refine and revise your methods over time.
Periodically undertake an audit. Be prepared to pare away any non-essential items. There is always a hierarchy of needs at any given time; be mindful of this and consider cost versus benefit.
7. You become good at coaching by coaching.
Take every opportunity to put yourself in front of athletes. If at the outset the available opportunities are unpaid, the value of experience you accumulate as a result is nevertheless worth the time investment.
8. Presence cannot be faked but it can be cultivated.
In Māori culture in New Zealand the term 'mana' describes possessing natural authority or presence. This a trait certain individuals possess as an intrinsic quality. However, in

those individuals who demonstrate even a hint of this quality it can be cultivated. Many of the best coaches are introverts and introspective by nature, but have developed their coaching persona over time by stepping outside of their comfort zone on a daily basis.

9. Act with conviction when in front of athletes.

A coach or practitioner who appears unsure or ill at ease does not inspire confidence. There is a place for questioning yourself, but this is not it.

10. Never underestimate what you have yet to learn.

In the previous chapter we introduced the 'instant expert' phenomenon. This is an extension of a well-established 'Dunning-Kruger' effect, whereby the less experienced (and more clueless) somebody is the more likely they are to underestimate what they don't know and overestimate their own competence.

11. It isn't just what you say.

The energy you bring each day, your body language and behaviours are critical to the environment you create.

12. Evolve your own style of coaching.

Over time you might adopt practices or even behaviours from working with and observing other coaches and practitioners; however do not imitate. Your own style must be entirely that.

13. Coach like Bruce Lee.

Martial arts legend Bruce Lee was an advocate of a style without a style, breaking free of a rigid and stylised approach. Be adaptable and fluid in your approach when instructing or communicating with athletes, to meet the needs of the situation and the individual.

14. Planning is important, but don't be wedded to the plan.

Athletes are biological organisms – a spreadsheet approach clearly cannot account for the host of different factors at play. Be prepared to adapt the plan – or go to plan B – according to how the athlete presents on any given day.

15. Make sure your session plan affords you the freedom to try things.

Play some jazz. The ideas that occur spontaneously during a session is where the magic happens.

16. Take every opportunity to add to your tool box.

The broadest array of skills and expertise you have at your disposal the better. Conversely, as the old adage goes, if you only have a hammer you will see and treat everything as a nail.

17. Expose yourself to as many sports as possible.

Once more these experiences in other environments are invaluable to provide different contexts for your practice. The ability to apply what you do with different sports and types of athlete is a critical skill to cultivate. There will also often be lessons to take and practices that can be adapted and applied to whatever sport(s) you end up working in.

18. Actively seek and pursue opportunities to step outside your comfort zone.

This is an important discipline and applies throughout your career, but it is all the more important when starting out. During the early stages in your journey particularly the comfort zone is the last place you should find yourself in; very little growth or learning happens there.

19. Park your ego at the door each day.

Failure to manage your ego can be the biggest barrier to your ongoing development and can ultimately be harmful to the athletes you serve.

20. You must earn the right every day.

Working with athletes and being involved in elite sport is a privilege. Much like an unjustified ego a sense of entitlement is among the worst traits a young coach or practitioner can demonstrate.

21. Practice self-awareness.

Engage in regular and unflinching self-reflection. The better you know yourself and the more honest you are the quicker you will overcome barriers and develop as a practitioner (and as a person).

22. Be good with humans and animals.

Being highly skilled and knowledgeable is ultimately futile if you are not able to successfully interact with athletes and others. There is a case to be made that any member of support staff regardless of specialism has no business dealing direct with athletes if they lack the emotional intelligence to do so.

23. Be authentic.

Athletes, much like kids and animals can tell if you are not fully invested or genuine in how you act and what you say.

24. It is not about you.

If your involvement in elite sport is driven by a desire for reflected glory or your principal motivation is your own advancement then at best you are a passenger and at worst a parasite.

25. Get a life.

Take steps to ensure that you have a life and interests outside of work. The greater perspective this affords you is invaluable.

Section Four – Tools for the Journey

Reflective Practice with Teeth – Asking the Hard Questions

Willingness to challenge and readiness to being challenged represent critical traits for elite practice. True reflective practice is predicated upon a readiness to ask yourself the hard questions. Not only that, we must resist deluding ourselves and answer the hard questions in an honest fashion. To develop requires stepping out of our comfort zone. Becoming better requires being unflinching in our self-assessment and reflection. In reality, despite the best intentions the majority pay lip service to this; it is easier (and far more comforting) to lapse into telling ourselves falsehoods or half-truths. It is important to recognise that you are your most important ally in this process, but you are also the biggest potential obstacle. Ultimately, for the process to elicit meaningful change, self-evaluation and reflective practice must have teeth. As a coach, practitioner, or indeed athlete, if we truly aspire to being elite we must be unflinching in asking and answering the critical questions, no matter how unpalatable the truths you uncover may be.

Before we begin, let us state at this outset that this chapter was written with the clear intention of being provocative. The objective is to challenge the reader; to prompt you to hold up a mirror to your motivations, your intentions and your actions. This chapter was not written with comfort in mind; indeed discomfort is integral to growth. Nevertheless, a disclaimer may be called for: if you are easily affronted, perhaps do not read on from here. For those that remain, courage...

THE ITERATIVE TERROR OF WHY...

The bronze medal for most discomfiting question for most coaches or practitioners is awarded to a simple and seemingly innocuous question: 'Why?'. The second most discomfiting is in fact a follow-up question to the first: 'Why?'. And, you guessed it, the hardest of all to deal with is when 'why?' is asked a third time.

The 'five whys' is a well-established technique for interrogating the truth about people's underlying thinking and motivations. In reality, three iterations of 'why?' is typically sufficient – and is often enough to reduce the unsuspecting coach or practitioner to a quivering wreck...

WHAT IS YOUR 'WHY'...

What motivates your practice? Where do you look for validation? How do you derive satisfaction? Is your mission genuinely athlete support, or is it a quest for reflected glory?

KNOW YOUR AUDIENCE...

Who do you ultimately feel accountable to? Those who pay you? Or the athletes you serve? Do your day to day actions really reflect your answer?

FEELING INVOLVED AND IMPORTANT...

What determines the extent of your involvement with an athlete at a given point in time? Genuine necessity? Self-importance? Self-interest?

OWNED OR BORROWED...

How did you acquire your philosophy? Was this a process of discovery and reasoning? Or did you simply adopt a ready-made philosophy or system of practice? Are you a follower or acolyte of a renowned 'authority' in your field of practice? Do you follow the tide of popular opinion on 'best practice'? Or do you take your own path?

BUILDING ON SAND OR CONCRETE...

What is the basis of your philosophy and practice? To what degree does convention and dogma feature?

DIGGING DEEPER...

What is the depth of your understanding? Have you drilled down to the foundations? Do you understand the concept down to first principles? Have you interrogated and tested the logic of the underlying premise and assumptions?

AN ANSWER FOR EVERYTHING...

Do you have all the answers? Do you really? Are you prone to exceeding the breadth and depth of your knowledge when counselling athletes? Do you fall prone to the 'Dunning-Kruger' effect*? Are you an instant expert**?

*Read more about the 'Dunning-Kruger' phenomenon in relation to confidence and competence in the next chapter

** 'Instant Expert' phenomenon: having read something somewhere, heard a podcast, attended a workshop, or observed practice, then immediately presents themselves as an authority on the topic

FIELD OF VISION...

How is your breadth of knowledge? Does your thinking, understanding, and perspective extend beyond your domain? Are you a specialist? Generalist? Both?

FRAME OF REFERENCE...

Do you know what 'elite' practice really looks like? Have you been exposed to a truly world-class environment? Would you know it if you saw it?

KNOWLEDGE IN CONTEXT...

How do you rate your knowledge of a given topic, versus your applied understanding of how it relates to practice? Do you understand it in context? Are you able to separate how the concept is presented in a textbook, versus how things work in practice?

NAVIGATING INFORMATION AND OPINION...

Do you truly exercise critical thinking? To practice critical thinking by definition you must first entertain alternative or opposing ideas: do you truly evaluate all the available evidence? Do you entertain the idea that your preconceived ideas might be wrong, or your pet methods may be flawed? Or do you simply gravitate towards evidence or opinions that support what you believe?

THE PERSONNEL OF YOUR INNER CIRCLE...

Who do you surround yourselves with? Who do you choose to populate your circle, professionally and personally? From whom do you seek feedback? With whom do you debate ideas? Look around yourself: do you see people who challenge you?

FOLLOWING THROUGH...

Words or actions? To what extent does one reflect the other? Do you fully consider the stakes when you commit to doing something, or pledge to take a course of action? How readily do you lapse? Do you fully appreciate the consequences and the damage to your credibility when you fail to fulfill a commitment, or honour your pledge?

STANDARDS...

What standards do you accept of yourself and others? Do you truly maintain and enforce these standards? If we are defined by the standards we accept of ourselves and others, what does this mean for you?

THE CRUNCH...

What price your integrity? In the crucible of a high-pressure environment, under challenge, or in difficult circumstances, do you remain true to yourself and your principles?

IN CLOSING...

Congratulations to those who made it to the end of this chapter! Your courage and readiness to expose yourself to the hard questions will be their own reward, particularly if you are able to answer in a frank and honest manner. Holding up a mirror up to ourselves, our motivations, our processes and practice is an important discipline for all practitioners. Those of us in the privileged position of working with athletes must recognise and respect the responsibility involved.

As we will explore in a later chapter, elite practice is not complicated; but elite practice is not easy. Practicing a growth mind-set and taking the necessary steps to hold ourselves accountable are necessary commitments if our practice is to evolve, and if we are to remain worthy of the faith placed in us.

Upholding Our Own Standards — Principles, Practices, and Process

After I first shared the original content that featured the 'hard questions' which appear in the previous chapter I subsequently met up to discuss these ideas with a coach I greatly respect named Dale Stevenson. Dale is best known as the coach of Tom Walsh, the recent Shot Put World Champion from the 2017 World Athletics Championships. Dale said he much enjoyed the 'hard questions for coaches' post I had shared, and he then asked me a very insightful question that I have deliberated upon much since our conversation. The question Dale asked was how do I make sure that I myself am held accountable to the 'hard questions'. In this chapter I attempt to provide an answer, and suggest some principles, practices and processes that we can use to keep ourselves honest and on track in our quest to be better.

STANDARDS DEFINE US...

We are defined by the standards we accept of ourselves and others. It is often easy to judge others by the high standards we aspire to. That said, it is more challenging and certainly less comfortable to hold those around us to account, and to do so in a constructive manner. This is the topic of a later chapter on accountability that appears in the next section.

For now we will focus the discussion on the process of holding ourselves accountable to standards of practice and behaviours.

Metacognition essentially concerns our knowledge and appreciation of our own thinking, reasoning, and problem-solving processes. In particular, metacognition comes into play when evaluating ourselves and holding ourselves to a standard of practice.

THE PARADOX OF PERCEIVED COMPETENCE...

> "Ignorance more frequently begets confidence than does knowledge..."
>
> – Charles Darwin

The seminal work by Justin Kruger and David Dunning [16] on the topic of metacognition and our ability to objectively and accurately evaluate our own competence provides something of a road map to avoid falling prey to what has become known as the 'Dunning-Kruger effect'.

The central tenet of the 'unskilled and unaware of it' phenomenon is that those who are demonstrably the least competent in a group grossly overestimate their abilities relative to others in the group [16]. Thus we see a paradoxical relationship whereby the most inept are also the least aware of their own ineptitude, and more likely to demonstrate (unfounded) confidence in their own competence.

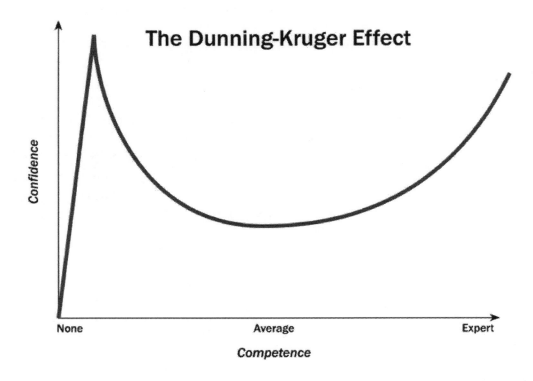

Figure 2 The Dunning-Kruger Effect

READINESS TO FACE REALITY...

The converse of the Dunning-Kruger effect is that a sign of true expertise is an ability to objectively and critically appraise one's own competence. By extension, it follows that those who possess genuine experience and expertise will more readily appreciate and acknowledge the complexity and uncertainty of the context in which we operate.

Scott Drawer was kind enough to write the foreword for my most recent textbook *Comprehensive Strength and Conditioning* [17]. Scott is a leader in innovation who has helped redefine the boundaries of best practice across an array of sports, and is one of the great free thinkers working in elite sport today. The wisdom he chose to share is that 'the true definition of an expert is somebody who recognises how much they don't know'.

SELF-AWARENESS AND HUMILITY...

I quoted Dan Pfaff in a previous chapter on the theme of ego in coaching. The salient point Dan made was that as long as a coach is capable of being honest with themselves the day to day experience of coaching athletes provides ample cause for humility (so that ego is not an issue). The point that can be lost with this piece of wisdom is that the decisive factor is whether we are capable of honesty.

From a long-term growth perspective, the most important trait for any practitioner to possess is self-awareness. The ability to be honest with oneself is arguably the best predictor of whether a practitioner has the propensity to develop and attain an elite level of practice.

Not only must an individual have a propensity for self-awareness, they also need to possess the will to exercise it. There is some indication that the 'unskilled and unaware of it' phenomenon may in part be wilful. In essence, the argument is that those who are inept have a motivation to ignore any evidence to this fact in order to protect against the challenge to their own self-concept [18].

When I encounter a young practitioner who is unsure of themselves this does not give me pause; this is something we can work with. What is an absolute red flag is a young coach who is over-confident and blind (perhaps wilfully) to what they do not know. In the absence of a major attitude adjustment, the latter represents somebody who is beyond help, and arguably unworthy of it.

Fundamentally, self-awareness and an accompanying willingness to turn a critical eye upon oneself are both critical to an individual's ability to learn and develop over time.

TOOLS FOR SELF-DIRECTED DEVELOPMENT...

Returning to how we might avoid an unaware state of incompetence, Kruger and Dunning [16] identify some key practices or 'meta-cognitive skills'. These skills or cognitive capabilities relate to the processes of assessing or evaluating ourselves, monitoring, comprehension, and recollection.

It follows that practicing this disciplines should allow us to retain the capacity to objectively rate our own performance, and thereby provide us with the means to remain on track and continue to progress.

CALIBRATING SELF-APPRAISAL...

Less competent individuals underestimate the capabilities of those around them and often grossly overestimate their own abilities, so that the very worst performers still estimate themselves to be above average [16]. Perhaps a lesson here is to be less dismissive and recognise the expertise of colleagues and peers more readily. Equally we should exercise a high level of scrutiny when evaluating how we rate ourselves.

Holding ourselves to a higher standard will certainly provide a stimulus for growth, as long as we embrace it in a positive manner, and view our perceived shortcomings as opportunities to be better.

In this spirit, we should seek out those who have observed our practice first-hand – including the athletes we coach. The external perspectives provided can provide an invaluable reference for comparison, assuming they are able to provide us with a frank and honest appraisal of our practice. The insights provided by a third party can prompt us to re-evaluate our self-appraisal where we find consistent discrepancies in the respective ratings on a particular element of our practice.

When it comes to rating our own abilities, with the best performers the obverse finding to what we have described previously is often observed. Specifically, the best performers have a tendency to underestimate their abilities, both in absolute terms and relative to their peers. Perhaps this reticence to score ourselves highly is important to avoid becoming complacent. Equally, input from an independent observer can provide affirmation and encouragement.

Competence is not only reflected in how we fare in accurately appraising our own abilities, but also our readiness to reappraise when presented with new evidence and differing perspectives.

FRAME OF REFERENCE...

Clearly it is necessary to have a valid frame of reference in order to gauge the level at which we are presently operating. The insights gained from observing world class operations are also important to inform what steps are necessary to progress our practice, and to ultimately ascend to elite level.

One of the biggest challenges for a practitioner who aspires to world class practice is gaining an appreciation of what true world class looks like. Much like 'elite' and 'high performance', the labels of 'world class' or 'world-leading' are often misapplied. Due diligence is therefore needed to seek out genuine world class practice, as opposed to an individual or set up that falsely proclaims themselves to be so.

We must therefore seek out opportunities to observe genuine world class practice. Ultimately this will require the investment to travel and spend time in these environments, in order to gain real insights into the processes and practices that differentiate world class operations.

STRESS TESTING WHAT WE KNOW...

First step is to articulate our approach and what underpins it. This process in itself helps to organise our thinking and dig deeper into the reasoning that underpins it.

We must be ready to expose these ideas to daylight and expose our thinking to scrutiny. On a day to day basis we should be open and receptive to questioning. When athletes and colleagues pose questions this challenges us to consider things more deeply in order to formulate an answer. Equally when we cannot summon a good answer or a strong case in support we are prompted to expand our knowledge and perhaps rethink our position.

Discussing our ideas with others can be a great way of challenging our thinking and deepening our understanding on a particular topic. Having people in our circle who we respect and are able to discuss our ideas with is invaluable. Equally, we should recognise that it is human nature to gravitate towards like-minded individuals. We should therefore intentionally seek out those with differing perspectives.

We might even consider sharing our thoughts in an open forum to expose our thinking to a wider and more diverse audience. The specific objective here is to invite questioning and external perspectives. Clearly this does require some bravery, and a certain tolerance for criticism.

KEEPING RECORDS...

Another cognitive bias to be mindful of, and take steps to guard against, is recall bias. We can be selective in what we recall, and the accuracy of our recollection may also not be what we think it is. Clearly the most straightforward way to combat recall bias is to maintain an objective record that we can refer to.

Practically, whilst we have a training plan, we should also keep a detailed log of sessions, sets and repetitions, to record what portion of the planned sessions were actually completed. These records will allow us to cross-reference our plans against the training that was actually logged; this will provide a more complete and accurate picture, for use during reviews, debriefs, and future plans.

To hold ourselves further accountable, we might consider adding another layer. For instance, we might keep a record of critical events and what decisions were taken. The 'decision diary' concept has been proposed and employed successfully in different realms (notably investment and finance), as tool to aid rational thinking and disciplined decision-making.

I readily admit I am presently quite poor at record keeping, and this is certainly an area for improvement. If we are able to be diligent and disciplined in this endeavour, this will provide an objective basis for reflection, rather than relying solely on the scope and accuracy of our recollection.

MOVING FORWARDS...

A host of metacognitive skills come into play in each part of the process on our journey to become better. Self-awareness and humility essentially underpin everything; these traits are required from the outset to appreciate the scope and complexity of the task we face. Moving forwards these same qualities are integral to the ongoing processes of assessing ourselves and monitoring our progress.

We can enlist the help of others to help calibrate our self-appraisal and provide external feedback of our progress. Once again, accepting constructive feedback is contingent upon humility and a readiness to be honest in our reflection; ultimately this will determine our ability to take this information on board and apply it to make the necessary changes.

As we have discussed there are a variety of strategies and tools we can employ to be systematic in our approach to becoming better. Practicing these metacognitive skills and developing them over time will derive real benefits on the ongoing journey towards elite practice.

Finally, in order to stay on the path we need to acknowledge that it is beguilingly easy to lapse into complacency and indulge in self-delusion. Therefore our success in utilising these principles and processes to raise our standards and achieve meaningful improvement over time will ultimately depend on our continued readiness to put our ego aside in order to hold ourselves accountable.

Practitioner Health – Making Practice in Elite Sport Sustainable

In the spheres of performance science much attention is paid to 'athlete health'. It has become widely recognised that lifestyle factors are critical, not only mediating performance and training adaption, but also impacting upon injury and illness. Despite such growing awareness, until very recently the notion of coach or practitioner health has not been widely considered in the same way. For the first time, important discussions on the topics of coach and practitioner health are being held more widely. For instance, 'coach health' in the field of strength and conditioning has been the recent topic of various podcasts and posts shared online. These discussions have raised important issues in relation to the unique challenges presently faced by practitioners operating in the Information Age. In addition to exploring these issues in more depth in this chapter, more importantly we will explore some strategies and tools to negotiate these challenges and ultimately find a way of working that is sustainable in the long term.

THE SINK OR SWIM EXISTENCE OF THE ASPIRING PRACTITIONER...

A survey conducted in 2016 by the UK Strength and Conditioning Association highlighted the plight of a large proportion of its members. This report made for very uncomfortable reading for those in the strength and conditioning profession. In particular, these findings drew attention to some stark realities and the struggles faced by a huge number of those seeking gainful employment in the field.

To a large extent these struggles stem from the over-saturated nature of the job market in the performance sciences and the field of strength and conditioning in particular. The reality is that the opportunities for paid work in elite and professional sport are very few.

Academic institutions in the UK particularly must take a huge chunk of the blame for continually fuelling this over-supply in the face of such limited demand. Yet the interest among school-leavers in pursuing sports sciences, and the prospect of a career in strength and conditioning in particular, remains undiminished. Whatever the moral arguments, in the face of such a ready source of revenue, universities and colleges will inevitably continue to offer increasing numbers of degree programmes, churning out more and more graduates into an already over-saturated pool.

Such unfavourable odds are not the only challenge faced by those starting out. The capricious nature of recruitment in professional sport and 'high performance' organisations such as national institutes of sport is another reality faced by those who aspire to work in sport. It is an unlovely fact of life that in many instances the recruitment process for athlete support positions (if a process is followed at all) is very far from being a meritocracy.

CHALLENGES FOR ALL...

We should note here that such challenges are not unique to the field of physical preparation. For instance, those who work in sports physiotherapy and associated therapy professions in professional sport are commonly expected to work long hours and often seven-day weeks, with little respite for much of the year. Sports coaches involved with different sports likewise face huge challenges in simply making an income from coaching, particularly in the case of 'amateur sports', such as track and field athletics, where being a volunteer coach is considered somehow 'noble'.

Therefore coaches and all practitioners working in sport face two fundamental challenges. The first is making working in sport viable as a way of making a living. In turn, the second challenge is finding a way to make this work practically in a manner that is sustainable in the long term. It is this second challenge that we will attempt to tackle here.

CLIMBING THE GREASY POLE...

Against this background the pressures faced by those fortunate enough to secure gainful employment in the field are considerable. Having managed to climb the 'greasy pole' and secured a much coveted paid position, the practitioner must then turn their attention to staying atop this perch. The perceived threat of losing out on such an opportunity to one of the masses below eagerly waiting any slip can seem very real.

One might argue that it is good thing that those who secure a paid position cannot lapse or become complacent. However, adopting such a defensive mind-set that is essentially driven by perceived threats to their position is not a healthy way of working.

Notable voices in the field have made a compelling argument that the major driver for the practices among strength coaches employed in college sport and the professional ranks is in fact fear. More specifically, many strength coaches are essentially adopting the methods, equipment, and practices that their competitors are using simply because they fear the consequences of not being seen to do so. Clearly fear is not a healthy source of motivation; certainly it is not conducive to a growth mind-set.

REAL AND IMAGINED PRESSURES...

Those working in professional sport, or indeed employed in any capacity in sport, will be familiar with the perceived pressure to be seen to be present. It is often viewed as a badge of honour for ambitious young practitioners particularly to be seen to be first in every morning and last to leave the facility each night.

Whilst they might be motivated by laudable intentions, such misguided demonstrations of commitment to the cause are often ultimately detrimental to the individual. In particular, investing such an amount of time each day in simply 'being at work' will inevitably be to the detriment of the individual's life and relationships outside work.

Aside from the hardships and unfavourable odds faced by those starting out, the dangers of burning out for those who do secure employment have recently been brought to the fore. Notable figures in the field, including Brett Bartholomew have spoken on the topic and introduced the concept of 'coach health' to a wider audience. Others such as Jorge Carvajal have highlighted the need to consider 'coach longevity', and have spoken publicly about their personal experiences in this regard to raise awareness of this important issue.

WORK-LIFE BALANCE IN ELITE SPORT...

It has been argued that in the realms of elite sport work-life balance is a myth. The contention of ideas such as the 'four burner theory' is that in order to achieve elite practice you must divert your energies away and essentially neglect other areas in your life (for example, friends, family), at least for periods of time.

Whilst being involved in elite sport inevitably involves trade-offs, particularly at critical times, I do not entirely subscribe to these views. Rather, balance can be maintained at different times simply by shifting the fulcrum on the seesaw, according to the priority area(s) at any particular time.

Adopting a humanist approach in our interactions with athletes is crucial to effective practice, particularly during pressure situations such as major competition, as we will explore in a later chapter. By definition this first requires being a viable human away from the workplace. On this basis alone I would argue that maintaining key relationships with family and friends outside of 'work' is in fact critical to being effective as a practitioner.

THE HUMAN ELEMENT OF PROFESSIONAL DEVELOPMENT...

Many practitioners who enthusiastically engage in professional development nevertheless often neglect to consider that logically this should also include developing themselves as a human. We need to recognise the value and importance of investing in developing ourselves beyond the realms of our professional practice.

Whatever the field of expertise, one's effectiveness as a practitioner is ultimately contingent on the quality and success of human interactions. From this viewpoint, failing to attend to this critical 'human element', and invest appropriate time in developing these areas, would appear to be negligent in the extreme.

There is an argument that in order to be a good coach it is necessary to first be a good human. Certainly to be a well-adjusted human, an individual's self-concept should be about more than merely their vocation as a practitioner. Successfully maintaining a life outside work is an integral part of developing who you are beyond the context of the sport or profession you work in.

At the very least, most would agree that when counselling athletes on lifestyle factors the message will be far better received if the practitioner is able to demonstrate personal success in these areas.

To paraphrase Mahatma Ghandi, to be credible when advocating certain healthy behaviours concerning sleep, dietary practices, and lifestyle in general with our athletes, the practitioner must be the change they wish to see.

As part of investing time in their personal development, coaches and practitioners should explore strategies to better negotiate the challenges of modern living. Given the pressures of elite sport, and associated demands on practitioners' time, adopting appropriate strategies will be all the more necessary in order to reclaim time and 'head space' to have some semblance of a life beyond work. As we will discuss, the pervasive nature of mobile technology and social media add new challenges that have not been faced previously. Such features of modern life and the Information Age therefore requires evolving new strategies and countermeasures.

CONTACT WITH THE OUTSIDE WORLD...

From a broader perspective, carving out time and investing energy in one's life beyond work should be viewed as a necessary countermeasure for combating the myopia that comes from residing in the bubble of elite sport. It is vitally important to be able to maintain some level of detachment and perspective. Retaining the sense that there is a real world outside of the bubble of the particular sporting context will serve the practitioner particularly well in the high-pressure situations around competition that are experienced in the crucible of elite sport.

To give an example, the best coach that I have worked with in professional sport is Brendan Venter. Brendan is hugely passionate about the game. However, Brendan is also a medical doctor; as such he has a profound understanding of what 'life and death' actually entails. Those fortunate to work with Brendan will attest to the fact this is evident in how he conducts himself, particularly during high-pressure situations. I recall a particular team talk in the changing room immediately following a bitterly disappointing loss in a vital game: rather than being caught up in the emotion of the moment, Brendan instead reassured the players that the sun would still rise the next morning. The broader perspective from Brendan's life beyond sport made this extraordinary display of leadership possible.

Conversely, in the absence of a life outside work, the only social interaction available to the practitioner is with colleagues and even the athletes with whom they work. This is a problem, as lines are likely to become blurred as a result. Clearly if our only social interaction is with our athletes, this is not conducive to maintaining professional boundaries. It is critical for both coaches and practitioners to maintain appropriate distance, in order to remain objective and conduct their duties effectively.

Moreover, solely interacting with others within the 'bubble' certainly does nothing to foster a sense of perspective. We must recognise how readily we can find ourselves inhabiting an echo chamber.

STRATEGIES FOR STAYING AFLOAT....

In case taking care of one's health and psycho-social well-being for its own sake is not a sufficiently strong motivator, retaining a functional life outside work is also an integral part of being an effective and credible practitioner, as we have spoken about. What this ultimately comes down to is allocating appropriate time and attention to managing oneself, in the same way as we do for our athletes.

A first step is having the bravery to resist the need to be seen to be present without any specific purpose. Once this obstacle is overcome, we can turn our attention to implementing strategies to be productive versus simply being busy.

Achieving success in this regard will involve being intentional and very deliberate in how we approach our work. Practically, this might include adopting simple measures such as batching admin tasks together and tackling them in a serial and a concentrated fashion, rather than breaking away to attend to other tasks as they come up, and being forced to repeatedly switch attention back and forth in between.

Ultimately we want to ensure we are actually being productive during the time we spend at the workplace each day. Once our work is done for the day, or we are no longer productive, we should then leave. Moreover, it is incumbent upon us to exercise the discipline to actually leave work when we leave work.

MANAGING CONSUMPTION...

Outside of day-to-day tasks, practitioners also face challenges in their efforts to engage in continuing education and professional development. As discussed in a previous chapter, chief among these is how to navigate the seas of information, particularly the vast quantities of data from a myriad of sources available online, in order to derive value and engage in meaningful learning.

A good analogy for the Information Age is the obesity epidemic in the developed world. The root cause is our compulsive behaviour and failure to make good choices in the face of ready access. Burgeoning obesity is simply the cumulative effect of the fact that as a population we ingest too many calories and too many of the calories we consume are short on nutritional value.

There are clear parallels here on how we consume data, and particularly how we utilise mobile technology to do so. In this era of 'hyper-connectivity' there is too much constant snacking and compulsive over-consumption of social media and the various other information sources available online. In general, we are continually attempting to ingest more bytes of data, and too many of the bytes of data we consume are short on meaningful information.

Clearly there is a need to be more selective. The sources of data we choose to consume each day must be carefully chosen to be rich in quality content. That said, arguably the bigger issue, and a critical first step, is that the way in which we consume this data must also become more directed and more deliberate.

Undirected or poorly directed sampling from this sea of information consumes vast quantities time and attention with very little return on investment. With unflinching self-reflection many of us would admit to being guilty of this. It is important that we understand what drives this behaviour. Often it is fear: fear of missing out; fear of becoming out of touch and no longer being on the cutting edge; and most of all fear that our peers in the field are gaining on us as a result.

A compounding factor is that smart devices and the software applications on these devices are likewise designed with the specific intent to foster, reward and reinforce the compulsive use of this technology. In this way, users of this smart technology are unwittingly the subject of 'operant conditioning'. Our attention becomes hostage and our behaviour becomes shaped by these devices.

Aside from becoming a slave to your smartphone, the modern phenomenon of smart devices and hyper-connectivity also blurs the boundaries between office hours and leisure time.

It is critical that we become aware of such triggers for compulsive and unproductive behaviours. We must also be mindful of what such behaviour costs us with respect to time that could be allocated to being productive, or invested in our health and relationships. Moreover, this recognition needs to be accompanied by action: we must take active steps to be more deliberate and intentional with how we use tools like mobile technology.

When seeking to develop in a professional capacity, relevant information must be consumed in such a way we can process and derive meaning. Only in this way will our efforts serve to ultimately improve our understanding or give us something we can actually use.

One practical measure is to look for resources that synthesise information from multiple sources. Another strategy is to find a mentor who is able to demystify, translate, provide meaning, and put the information in context in a way that makes it real and applicable.

TAKE TIME TO GO OFFLINE...

Finally, and perhaps most importantly, we must take steps to 'go offline' when not at work. In a landmark case for occupational health, the right to disconnect from receiving and responding to work communications outside of office hours was recently mandated in law in France. As practitioners, we must follow this lead and reach agreement with colleagues (and athletes) to clearly define and maintain 'work hours', on the understanding that we will not respond to communications outside of those hours.

Clearly this must be reinforced by the discipline to unplug from mobile devices and resist the impulse to check email and social media during these offline hours. Furthermore, the reclaimed time should be allocated and invested appropriately in health, relationships and cultivating a life outside work.

Part Two: For Coach and Leader

Section One – Philosophy

The Simplicity and Complexity Paradox

The concept of yin and yang is often illustrative and I return to this theme often when presenting on different topics, as the reader will notice in these chapters. In essence, yin and yang describes how opposing elements (light and dark, fire and water) paradoxically serve to complement and ultimately define each other. Much the same applies when considering simplicity versus complexity. There are many instances where each of these elements apply in the realms of coaching and various facets of practice in elite sport. In this chapter we will explore the paradoxical - or yin and yang - relationship between simplicity versus complexity in the fields of coaching, physical preparation and sports injury.

KEEP IT SIMPLE...

"Know your sport or event in its utter complexity so you can teach it simply"

— Greg Hull

There is a strong case for simplicity when it comes to coaching and instruction. As we spoke about in a previous chapter there are apparent benefits to being sparing and concise with the explicit instruction employed to steer an athlete's learning when acquiring new skills. Essentially, the less cognitive 'noise' or baggage that accompanies the learning process, the more robust the skill is likely to prove under pressure.

From this viewpoint, capturing the essence of the movement to keep things as simple as possible when introducing new concepts and movement skills has clear advantages. Finding ways to relate new skills to what the athlete already knows is one tactic that allows the amount of 'new' information during the learning process to be kept to a minimum.

"If you cannot explain it simply you do not understand it well enough"

— Albert Einstein

THE CURSE OF FACILE SOLUTIONS...

So if simplicity is so valuable in teaching and learning, does this mean that by definition the simplest solution is always the best?

Clearly this will depend somewhat on the situation, but in short, the answer is typically 'no'. Herein lies the paradox.

"For every complex problem there is an answer that is clear, simple, and wrong"

— H.L. Mencken

Most coaches and practitioners will be familiar with the scenario of a brash young upstart who thinks they have cracked it and that they possess the solution to fix every problem. Essentially if you only have a hammer in your toolbox, the likelihood is that you will see everything as a nail. This folly is beguiling and the only known cure is acquiring deeper knowledge and experience.

Indeed, if we are honest with ourselves, it is likely that to some extent this scenario describes our younger selves, before sport and the complexity of biology and individual responses taught us a lesson.

ACKNOWLEDGING COMPLEXITY...

Irrespective of the area concerned, no single approach offers a panacea. There is no one universal remedy that applies in all scenarios or with all individuals.

We must acknowledge that we are dealing with complex adaptive systems. By definition, there will always be multiple factors in play. There is a need for a case by case approach. The situation is also be highly dynamic, so we cannot expect the same solution to apply at different points in time even for the same individual.

Looking beyond the athlete, if we factor in social dynamics and the human interaction elements inherent with the coach-athlete relationship and the wider support team, we encounter further layers of complexity. Over recent years progress has been made in reframing models of coaching with the aid of complexity theory, acknowledging the complex and multifaceted nature of a process that is built upon interaction and interpersonal elements [19].

The benefits of acknowledging complexity in how we approach athletic preparation are evident. As we will see in the next section, there are numerous examples of the superiority of multifaceted or 'complex' interventions over simple single-mode solutions.

IT'S ALL IN THE BLEND...

For instance, when training to develop the capability to express power, 'mixed methods' approaches generally show superior results in comparison to single training mode interventions [20]. Interestingly, the blended approach can also yield additional improvements that are not evident when the respective training modes are applied in isolation [21].

In the area of injury prevention, it is similarly evident that when respective approaches are employed in combination the outcomes are far more positive [22]. A consistent finding is that combined interventions are more effective than single mode interventions.

Indeed, investigations have reported that when the respective single interventions are employed in isolation they may fail to elicit the desired changes [23].

Once again, it is the blend or 'complex' of different approaches which is the factor that differentiates between successful versus unsuccessful outcomes.

YIN AND YANG...

To bring it all together, the yin of simplicity is balanced and complemented by the yang of complexity. Irrespective of the practitioner's area of specialism, both elements are likely to come into play in practice.

Simplicity is king when it comes to communicating ideas and less is certainly more when it comes to instruction. Complexity must however be embraced when considering each athlete and the situation at hand, in order to properly consider the problem and ultimately devise a solution. A complex of approaches is therefore generally the best approach when selecting (and blending) methods in coaching, training and treatment interventions.

The Olympic Pursuit of Inspiration

O ver the course of the Rio Olympic and Paralympic Games in 2016 there was much talk of inspiration. For instance, the BBC in the UK ran the feature 'Get Inspired'. In New Zealand it was 'Be The Inspiration', complete with an 'Inspiration Hub'. All of which, in a circular fashion, inspired this chapter on the topic of 'Inspiration'.

THE OTHER MEANING OF INSPIRATION...

For the most part, when those in the media talk of 'inspiration' or 'being inspired' they are referring to those watching sport being inspired to strive to achieve the feats that they have seen, or attempt to emulate their sporting heroes. In this way, great athletes are often described as 'an inspiration to others'. Essentially, this is inspiration borne of admiration – essentially the 'I want to be like them when I grow up' scenario.

The alternative meaning of inspiration - and the definition that this chapter will mostly focus on – considers inspiration in the sense of stimulating thought or inspiring new ideas.

BEING INSPIRED...

In spite of the controversy that blighted the lead up to the Rio Games and the revelations that continued throughout, as a coach and practitioner I was nevertheless inspired in this way by the Rio Olympics. Having returned to the UK I woke up in the early hours in order to watch the closing stages of the heptathlon and then the final of the men's 100m. When I returned to bed my mind was abuzz with thoughts and ideas, inspired by what I had just seen. Sleep was a long time coming.

And so sport, and a pinnacle event like the Olympics in particular, is in itself a source for inspiration in the sense of provoking thought and stimulating new ideas.

THE GENESIS OF IDEAS AND INNOVATIONS...

Seeking inspiration and creating an environment conducive to ideas and innovation is likewise always topical in the realms of elite sport, but particularly so in the afterglow of an Olympic cycle.

Returning to definitions, innovation is essentially reframing or reworking an existing concept or practice. Conversely the genesis of a new idea is that most rare of things. In the realms of physical preparation and athletic development if you are prepared to look deep enough and on a long enough timeline typically most 'novel' practices have in fact been seen before.

The quest for innovation and new ideas is a recurring challenge across the different branches of sports sciences, sports medicine and sports coaching. This applies both from a commercial viewpoint and for those in the field seeking the cutting edge (such as Team Sky and their mantra of marginal gains).

LIGHTNING RODS FOR IDEAS...

The genesis of new ideas and initiatives can be profoundly influenced by environment. This might simply be exposure to an individual who challenges and provokes thought. In this way, just one individual can be the source of inspiration; and this alone can create an environment that provides fertile soil and the stimulus for the growth of new ideas.

One common feature of such individuals who provide inspiration to those around them is that they are critical thinkers. However, beyond that also these individuals are also generally free thinkers who are unconstrained by convention. In essence, these are the people brave enough to pose the 'what if' questions.

RECEPTIVE AUDIENCE...

Being receptive to the inspiration afforded by such individuals in turn requires a mind that is not unduly troubled by such dangerous free thought. Possessing the necessary mental dexterity and agility of thought to take full advantage generally comes from the innate quality of being curious. Indeed curiosity alone is perhaps the single most important trait that those who merit the dubious title 'thought-leader' have in common with those who are inspired by these agents of change.

Aside from innate curiosity, the capacity to be receptive to 'being inspired' is without doubt aided immeasurably by being exposed to 'rainmaker' figures during the course of a career, particularly when starting out. In contrast, this capacity is likely to be stunted by organisations and high performance systems that seek to indoctrinate rather than inspire and encourage free thinking. This applies particularly to internship programmes, such as those offered by national sports institutes. Those who are a product of such systems can be institutionalised to the extent that they are immune or even averse to inspiration, and indeed free thought.

A hallmark of inspiration is that it is fleeting, and as such this necessitates a mind that is attentive and open to these rare 'light bulb' moments.

CONDUCIVE CONDITIONS...

Thoughts and ideas often come to me when I am traveling and have an abundance of time and space to think. Conversely, the routine of a normal work schedule seems to be less conducive. It is as though these thoughts and ideas are furtive and seem to hide away, only coming to the fore at the most random of times.

For instance, it is often when I wake up in the early hours and I don't get back to sleep straight away that thoughts come one after another. Once more, this occurs most often when I'm travelling - and jet lag is a co-factor here. The recent instance I mentioned earlier in the chapter of waking up to watch the Olympic 100-metre final in the early hours is a perfect example.

It may be that it is the something about the state of 'disconnection' – middle of the night, unfamiliar environment, different time zone – that facilitates ideas to come to the surface. And once again, it is necessary to be attentive and receptive to these fleeting moments of inspiration, even if they arise at an inconvenient time (and interfere with your beauty sleep).

RAINMAKERS I HAVE KNOWN...

Returning to the topic of lightning rods or 'rainmakers' who stimulate thought and provide the spark for those around them, I have been fortunate to have encountered a number of these individuals throughout the course of my career to date.

This first of these encounters came at the very start of my journey in elite sport, when my PhD research brought me into contact with Brendan Venter. That first preseason I spent with London Irish rugby club when Brendan had just taken the helm as Player/Coach I vividly recall returning home every evening buzzing with thoughts and new ideas. Indeed it was over these months and the subsequent two seasons that Brendan was in charge that I came up with many of the novel training interventions that eventually formed my PhD thesis.

Brendan is the epitome of the rainmaker individual described earlier. Brendan is a practicing medical doctor and boasts a fearsome intellect. As a coach, Brendan was (and remains) unconstrained by conventional wisdom and 'coaching manual' practice, as all of his coaching philosophies and methods are uniquely his own. I caught up with Brendan recently and he told me what motivated him to become involved in coaching in the first instance was his firm belief that it could be done better.

Brendan brought a great deal of knowledge and practical experience from his years playing at the top level to his coaching. Equally, and more uniquely, he was ready to entertain any idea or methodology and evaluate it on merit; if it stood initial scrutiny he tested it under field conditions, and what didn't pass was discarded. Brendan inspired and challenged the players and staff around him; indeed an astonishing number of the players from that era have since become successful coaches themselves.

This early exposure to such a bold and free thinker had a profound influence on my career as a practitioner and coach. In the years since I have been fortunate to encounter several other key figures who have provided inspiration and influenced both my thinking and practice.

To name a few, in his capacity as National Coach and Performance Director Roger Flynn relentlessly challenged me to explore different avenues to come up with new and better training solutions for players at different levels of the national programme during our time at Scottish Squash. I was still new to the sport when I met Roger; not only was he responsible for bringing to my attention the critical facets of the game, but more than that he actively encouraged me to bring a different lens and alternative perspectives from my work in other sports. What drove our practice was the notion that our programme would lead rather than follow, and Roger made sure we continued to push the boundaries and remain on the cutting edge.

Following my arrival in New Zealand I was then hugely fortunate to make the acquaintance of Angus Ross. Angus is not only a great mind, but a man of boundless curiosity whose fascination with sport and performance has been undiminished by his many years' involvement in elite sport and its administration. Angus brings genuine enthusiasm to his endless quest to find answers to real performance questions that come directly from his continuing involvement in the field of practice with athletes. Angus and I continue to regularly engage in 'what if' discussions spanning a random assortment of topics; Angus has been personally responsible for many of the ideas that have borne a host of PhD research in New Zealand over recent years (many co-supervised by Angus himself).

In the recent period I have been similarly fortunate to cross paths with Scott Drawer; in each of Scott's respective roles with UK Sport, the Rugby Football Union, and now Team Sky, he has been tasked with finding novel solutions and driving innovation and knowledge transfer to evolve best practice in the field. As such, Scott has a unique grounding on the process of cultivating new ideas and bringing innovation into practice.

Finally, at the end of last year I had the privilege to finally meet Dan Pfaff during a visit to Altis in Phoenix. As a track and field coach naturally I had followed Dan's work and teaching from afar for a number of years, and had even sought out those who had worked under Dan's mentorship. Meeting the man himself and sharing some time with him was an incredible experience. Throughout the week I spent in Phoenix my mind was once more buzzing with thoughts and ideas in a way that I hadn't known since that aforementioned period at the outset of my career. Dan is an extraordinary mind and is unique for a number of reasons, but perhaps most striking is his genuine desire to impart knowledge and share his insights with any coach or practitioner who wishes to learn. Rarer still is that this is borne of true altruism. Extraordinary indeed.

IN CLOSING...

And so concludes our exploration of the Olympic pursuit of inspiration. As you have read I have been fortunate meet certain individuals at different points in my career who possess the ability to inspire those around them to think and perhaps to dream. I hope to encounter more in the years to come. Moreover I hope to remain receptive to the inspiration afforded by sport and those involved in the pursuit of better, higher, faster. Light bulb moments may be occasional and fleeting; nevertheless they remain available for those who are open and attentive to them.

Nuance: The Path to Enlightenment in Athletic Preparation

Nuance is an under recognised keystone of practice in elite sport. We have spoken previously about critical thinking as a critical skill for coaches and practitioners in the Information Age, as a means to evaluate and integrate information from different sources. Nuanced understanding is equally critical for the steps that follow. Nuance is required to derive real meaning from the knowledge acquired and make use of it. Nuance is also critical to cope with the complexity inherent in human performance. In this chapter we will make the case for practicing nuance as an active skill in order to combat the epidemics of superficial knowledge and binary thinking.

PERILS OF THE AGE...

Just as with critical thinking, nuance has become more crucial and yet increasingly rare in the Information Age. Social media has become a prominent source of information for many coaches and practitioners. By its nature, the information delivered on these platforms is the condensed and bite-sized version; this is integral to what makes it useful. The inevitable downside is that this format does not lend itself to nuance.

Social media is a great tool for learning when used with intention, and with the acknowledgement that it skims the surface. It is our use of this tool that is the issue. We need balanced consumption. If social media is our predominant source of information this is 'fast food' learning. At best information consumed in this way yields superficial knowledge.

Nuance is also notably absent in the polarised debates on different topics on these platforms.

An associated trend is the extremism in the way that viewpoints are presented on social media platforms. Adopting an extreme or rigid position on a contentious topic has become a tactic to attract a following. Social media has also become a forum used to propagate a particular narrow world view or school of thought, and to attack others who express other views.

Sadly, this extremism is not only the domain of the ever-growing legion of 'virtual experts'. Those in the fields of sports science and sports medicine are increasingly guilty of dogmatic behaviour and unworthy conduct on social media. These platforms are increasingly vehicles for various agendas, be it commercial or self-interest (or some combination thereof).

VOICES OF REASON...

Amidst the ill-informed clamour on social media, there have been recent calls for reason from prominent voices in the applied sports sciences. Mike McGuigan wrote an excellent editorial [13] on the fallacy of extreme positions and polarised debates. The theme of the editorial was that context is critical, and inevitably 'it depends'.

It was likewise welcome and very reassuring that complexity and nuance were recurring themes in both the presentations and surrounding discussions during the high performance strength and conditioning symposium hosted at the United States Olympic Center in May 2017. This was perhaps a reflection of the level of professional experience and accumulated wisdom of those assembled for the event, which is great credit to the organisers.

ALL IS SPECTRAL...

> "I struggle with absolutes..."
>
> — Dan Pfaff

Absolutes are rare in the realms of human performance. Physics aside, there are very few universal rules. In general, it is generally unsafe to generalise.

Regular readers will be aware that I cite Dan Pfaff often. Nuanced understanding is a hallmark of coaching wisdom and once again Dan offers a perspective that resonates on this topic. Dan describes athletic preparation in terms of 'spectral phenomena' - i.e. existing on a spectrum.

Elite athletes are a special population. They are 'outliers'. Moreover athletes are also a diverse and heterogenous population. Each athlete sits in a different point on a continuum.

Diversity is acknowledged in many sports (notably team sports). But the continuum concept also applies to specialised events. A closer looks shows that athletes with differing individual profiles bring a range of solutions to the same problem. This persists even when we eliminate aspects of physiology and tactics.

An example from track and field athletics is that two high jumpers can clear the same height with radically different approach velocity and take off mechanics (exemplified by Donald Thomas versus Stefan Holm). Hence, in jump events athletes are often broadly classified as either a 'power-jumper' or a 'speed-jumper'. Once again, in reality each athlete sits on a different point on a continuum between these two poles.

Given the nature of what we are dealing with, it should not be surprising that exceptions are the rule.

COMPLEX VS COMPLICATED...

> "Make things as simple as possible. But not simpler."
>
> — Albert Einstein

The allure of absolutes and fixed mind-sets is the sense of (artificial) certainty it creates. Such need for reassurance stems from the fact that the alternative to the binary view of the world seems to involve too many questions and complications. Opening ourselves up to the possibility that there might be more to it (and it depends) is frightening to entertain. Allowing for such complexity could leave us lost at sea. Many choose not to be troubled by troubling possibilities.

Just as we crave certainty, we struggle with imperfection. In the face of critique we are too quick to discredit entirely. Observing that there are apparent flaws or questions raised too often leads us to disregard what has been presented entirely - and indeed many do not trouble themselves to entertain it in the first instance.

On the contrary there is almost always some merit whatever the limitations. We can find value if we remain open to looking. Equally we don't have to swallow anything whole. Again the situation is not binary. Which brings us back to nuance.

On a fundamental level we need to accept that everything (and everybody) is in its essence imperfect. Each piece of evidence that comes to light will inevitably be incomplete. There is always a need to interpret and to infer, in order for the information on offer to become 'actionable intelligence'. Absolutely it is important to acknowledge the flaws and shortcomings in whatever is presented. Equally, most often there is value to be found and lessons to be taken.

Complex does not have to be complicated. A nuanced understanding allows the complexity integral to the process of preparing athletes to be navigated. In this way we can find clarity.

IT DEPENDS...

The folly of dealing in absolutes becomes readily apparent when we expose ideas and practices to 'live' conditions and real-life athletes. Any concept too slavishly applied will inevitably be a wrong fit in certain conditions or circumstances, and for a number of the athletes we encounter.

We are dealing with complex adaptive systems. By definition, we must account for this complexity and be ready to adapt our approach to each athlete, and to the situation at hand.

By extension every statement should essentially be marked with a virtual asterix. We should accept as a given there will be a number of exceptions or caveats to be listed in the virtual footnotes.

The notion that 'it depends' is of course not generally well received by those craving certainty and facile answers to complex questions.

Instead of searching for straightforward and easy answers, we should perhaps switch our thinking to seek to define the parameters for the problem at hand, and establishing what factors we need to consider for each individual. To do so requires that we allow for nuance in our thinking, and accept that it will be a process of critical reasoning on a case by case basis.

COMPLEXITY AND CONTEXT...

The presumption that a universal rule exists is clearly nonsensical. So too is the assumption of uniformity. Diversity aside, even for the same individual the situation is highly dynamic.

A host of bio-psycho-social factors affect athlete's state at any given time affecting how they perceive, experience, and respond to a training stressor. By definition, these factors and thereby the athlete's state are in constant flux.

Peeling this back another layer, we must consider phenotype (expression of inherited traits) as an evolving picture. How an individual athlete responds will inevitably evolve over time.

For instance, prior exposure to training exerts a legacy effect [24]. In turn, this will alter how the athlete responds to the same training, year on year. There will also be a 'legacy effect' of the athlete's cumulative injury history. Once again, the residual effects and changes resulting from previous injuries will affect structural integrity, capacity, and capability to a varying degree as time goes on.

In addition to accounting for complexity at the level of the individual, nuance in relation to application extends to considering context and the situation at hand.

NEGOTIATING UNCERTAINTY...

As outlined there are a host of factors to consider in the reasoning process, and a need to allow for the fact that the situation is highly fluid and in constant flux. Moreover many of the aforementioned bio-pyscho-social factors and other elements at play are not completely knowable.

With wisdom acquired over time, coaches and practitioners can demonstrate a level of 'expert intuition', largely based on associations learned from many years of reflective practice. However, even the best and most experienced coach cannot entirely predict the outcome. Judgement is a matter of probabilities (there are few certainties). At any time there is also the possibility of a scenario we have not encountered before.

For other mortals, 'heuristics', or rules of thumb, can help guide our decisions during everyday practice. Equally, by definition these are approximations, and we need to acknowledge that our immediate impressions and snap judgements are prone to different sources of systematic error [25]. We should therefore temper our confidence accordingly and be ready to consider things more deeply and deliberately, particularly in the case of important decisions. Inevitably we are dealing in best guesses.

Armed with this understanding, coaching becomes an ongoing process of hypothesis testing. We take our educated best guess, observe, monitor outcome, alter approach or adjust course accordingly, (repeat).

BRINGING IT ALL TOGETHER...

We opened up this chapter with the statement that nuance is a keystone of practice in elite sport. As outlined, nuance must be applied in how we consume information in order to cope with imperfection, find value, and derive meaning. This is particularly vital when delving into the mire on social media.

Nuance as it relates to both understanding and application is required to implement knowledge acquired into practice under 'live' conditions and real athletes, with all the complexity, variety and variability this entails.

In closing, nuance is not only the path to enlightenment but also offers the means for enlightened practice.

Section Two – Systems and Teams

Defining 'Elite' in Sport

The term elite appears incessantly in the sporting domain. But what do we mean when we say elite? What does 'elite' mean to you? For many when the term 'elite' is used what this calls to mind is more akin to 'elitist'. The interpretation of 'elite' is often synonymous with 'exclusive', and a domain reserved for the chosen few. In this chapter we will dig a little deeper into these misconceptions and explore what differentiates elite from elitist. By the end of this discussion we hope to provide an outline of the hallmarks that constitute truly elite practice in sport.

ELITE IS A PRACTICE NOT A LABEL...

The harsh (and often surprising) reality is that the individuals and the level of practice that occur in sport at elite level are not 'elite' by default. As noted in a previous chapter, simply using labels such as 'high performance' (or 'elite') does not make it so. The term elite must be earned. Even at the top tier of competition in professional and Olympic sport there are critical elements that differentiate the truly elite.

What distinguishes elite practice at these lofty heights may appear subtle; however in the rare cases where a truly elite culture and environment is encountered, the difference in behaviours (and outcomes) is in fact remarkable.

ELITE ≠ ELITIST...

Firstly, and most importantly we must differentiate 'elite' from 'elitist'. Being elite does not equal being elitist. This is the single most common misconception with regards to elite practice. By extension, many of the issues with organisations and systems in sport arguably arise from confusing elite with elitist.

For instance, 'elite' does not automatically imply exclude. Elite behaviours and standards can be applied regardless of the level or group you're working with.

DIFFERENTIATING ELITE FROM ELITIST...

Elitist organisations favour the uppermost few; the 'best and brightest', as judged in accordance with the conventions of the institution. In reality most often what such systems reward are the best and most enthusiastic conformists, and marginalises and dispirits the rest.

When viewed in this way, it is easy to see how an elitist environment is contrary to promoting and developing the qualities that are required of a good coach and practitioner.

Compromise and conformity have no place in elite sport. Truly elite behaviours are underpinned by critical thinking and readiness to challenge.

In contrast to an elitist organisation, an elite team or leadership structure invites and gives credence to all voices regardless of rank. We will return to the topic of organisational structures and elite practice later in the chapter...

THE ELITE PATH IS NOT COMFORTABLE...

"The trick is that there is no trick..."

— Brendan Venter MD

Elite behaviours are not complicated. There is no trick. However, being elite does not afford the luxury of being comfortable.

The reality is that the day-to-day practice of being elite is hard and exacting work. Being elite involves constant challenge, unending questioning and unflinching evaluation. Elite practice also demands the highest standards; and holding oneself and others accountable to those standards.

Those who wish to be elite therefore must be ready to be uncomfortable. Practicing elite behaviours and upholding these standards on a daily basis may also not make you popular with colleagues and leaders (more on this later).

THE EXTRA MILE IS NEVER CROWDED...

Whilst there is nothing complicated about elite practice, it is hard graft and very little about it can be described as 'comfortable'. It is therefore easy to see why so few people stick to this path.

On the whole, it is far easier to conform. It is much less hassle to follow along without question, and in many instances this may improve your career progression. Even with the best intentions, it is also tempting and beguilingly easy to compromise standards; the immediate consequences of doing so are often minimal, and rarely will anybody call you on it (too much hassle). Anything for an easy life.

Adopting a different strategy and following an alternative path of hard work and discomfort requires a rare and special kind of person. As we see in the next section, in some instances this may be somebody who simply recognises that they do not possess the advantages necessary for the conventional route and so must seek alternatives.

WHEN THE CONVENTIONAL PATH IS NOT A VIABLE OPTION...

Just as necessity is the mother of invention it is also the catalyst for challenging convention in sport and exploring a different path. The absence of a viable alternative often provides the background for the convention-defying great leaps forward that periodically occur in sport.

As Malcolm Gladwell highlighted in his recent book David and Goliath [26] in many instances the individuals and teams who take these great leaps come from a position of disadvantage.

As Gladwell describes, agents of change are often underdogs who simply recognise the reality of they are faced with: their lack of advantages mean that following the conventional path will likely lead to defeat. In essence their situation is sufficiently desperate that they are prepared to entertain and pursue less comfortable alternatives.

The 'underdog as agent for change' scenario exemplifies that paradigm-shifting and ground-breaking practice in elite sport is far from the product of an elitist environment.

COMETH THE HOUR...

Returning once more to Malcolm Gladwell's writing, in *David and Goliath* Gladwell identifies that the hallmark of the entrepreneur and innovator is that they do not score high on 'agreeableness'.

An agreeable person generally seeks the approval of the group. Those who are agreeable are not inclined to offend people's sensibilities. As such, agreeable people do not often upset the apple cart, even if they do see things differently. After all doing so might risk an unfavourable reaction from peers and being ostracised from the group.

Ground-breaking practice therefore requires an individual who is not unduly troubled by such concerns. Those searching for elite levels of practice should therefore look to the maverick few who do not seek the approval of the group and are content to defy convention, even at the risk of being an outcast.

ORGANISATIONS AND ELITE PRACTICE...

In general, conventional organisations favour agreeable people. Managers naturally warm to unquestioning and compliant employees; after all they are so agreeable. Everybody loves a 'team player'.

There is a tension here between conventions in management versus what is required to be elite. Cutting edge practice demands rogue thinkers who do not score high on the agreeable scale. Conventional organisational structures, management practices and recruitment policies by their nature do not favour the very types of individual that are required for elite practice.

The true test of the calibre of a leader or system is how the individual or organisation entertains and responds to divergent thinking. It is important to clarify here that we are not talking about rebelliousness borne of contrariness, or acting up for the sake of it. Rather, we are referring to holding alternative views and genuine convictions.

On a positive note, there has been progress in recent times in our use of the term 'disruptive'. Previously 'disruptive' has generally had negative connotations, for example a 'disruptive' child at school. However increasingly 'disruptive' is being used in a positive sense. For instance, 'disruptive' is now commonly used to describe business models that have defied convention and 'broken the mould', achieving success by turning standard practice on its head.

DISCORD AND THE 'HIVE MIND'...

Let us consider our views on confrontation and challenge versus compromise and conformity. In most realms the latter are generally deemed more desirable. However, in the context of elite sport (and indeed an organisation in any field that aspires to cutting edge practice) this is absolutely not the case.

The urge or pressure to confirm to popular or dominant view of the group should be resisted at all cost. When we allow our thinking to fall under the influence of the group we effectively reduce our sample size or number of independent functioning minds contributing to reasoning process.

For the 'hive mind' of the group to work effectively it needs independent minds and diversity of views [27]. Practically this requires those who are capable of not only holding alternative views but also expressing these views regardless of outside pressures and influences. The wisdom of the hive mind is predicated upon strong individuals who can resist being easily influenced by the prevailing view or the dominant voice in the group.

From this viewpoint, conformity and compromise can be seen as afflictions that particularly affect those agreeable types who are most prone. A group populated with these types becomes an echo chamber, particularly in the face of a dominant personality.

To avoid 'group bias' that skews judgement and incapacitates the ability of the group to think rationally it follows that we should be recruiting and promoting strong independent minds. In essence we want those who are most able to resist collusion and retain the capacity to challenge 'group think'.

In other words to avoid systematic errors in judgement we need to accept dissonance and entertain dissenting voices. Indeed they should be praised for enriching the group with alternative and diverging views.

A ROUTE MAP TO 'ELITE'...

Organisations need to abandon elitism and the normal conventions of leadership and management if they are to be elite. Discard compromise, conformity, and take a dim view on agreeableness. Rather the culture should be built upon readiness to challenge and be challenged, a willingness to resist convention, and the ability to see things through a different lens.

Leaders need to recognise that challenge and even conflict are necessary precursors for elite practice. Rather than rewarding and recruiting those who parrot the right answers (elitist), the objective should be to seek those who ask the best questions (elite).

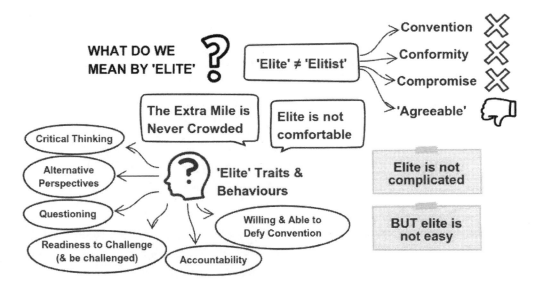

Figure 3: What do we mean by 'Elite'?

The true sign of a strong leader can be found in those they choose to surround themselves with. More specifically, what is most revealing is whether the 'inner circle' is populated by independent individuals who challenge the thinking of the leadership, or simply a collection of nodding dogs.

A FINAL THOUGHT…

We need to understand that the universal trend of regression towards the mean applies with elite teams, just as it does with everything else (hence universal). In the absence of periodic and timely intervention, any team or organisation will inevitably regress to a natural state of mediocrity.

There is an element of physics to this. Let us use the analogy of a balloon. To keep our balloon elevated above the ground will require us to give it impetus at regular intervals; otherwise it will come back down to earth, and settle on the ground among all the other self-proclaimed high performing balloons.

Achieving elite practice represents a challenge; maintaining practice at an elite level is another challenge entirely. With this in mind, it will be necessary to adopt and enforce appropriate countermeasures to prevent lapses. Not only do we need to guard against complacency, more pertinently we also need to be ready to put in the requisite work to 'maintain elevation'. Finally, the pervasive forces of 'group think' and convention need to be recognised and actively challenged at every turn.

Accountability – The Holy Grail for 'High Performance' Systems

Igh performance has become a buzz word that appears constantly in relation to sporting bodies worldwide and organisations associated with sport at all levels. The reason for the inverted commas ('High Performance') in the title is that this term has become so over-used and misused that it has arguably been rendered meaningless. Using the label does not make it so. In this chapter we discuss the elements that must be present in order for an environment and the practitioners who work in it to merit the title 'high performance'.

> "A significant degree of accountability must be established"
>
> — Phil Coles, Director of Performance and Medical at San Antonio Spurs

In a feature for the *leadersinsport* website Phil Coles, formerly of Liverpool Football Club (and others) and now working with NBA side San Antonio Spurs, attempted to define the key constituents of a 'high performance unit'. In this article Coles describes that the key objective in leading a high performance unit is ensuring the respective disciplines work together towards the common goal of improving performance. But Coles identifies that there must first be accountability.

NO PASSENGERS – ACCOUNTABLE TO WHAT?

Delving further into the notion of accountability, there is a need to determine what role each individual service provider providing 'high performance support' is actually playing in the process.

> "The success of the team as a whole will always be a consideration, but perhaps more importantly, objective markers should be set to monitor the success or otherwise in each of the individual processes introduced"
>
> — Phil Coles

TURKEYS DON'T VOTE FOR CHRISTMAS...

Government funded national sports institutes can be quite ruthless in holding the athlete, coach, and sport itself accountable. Consequences follow when athletes fail to perform to expected level during a season of competition or if the sport fails to meet performance targets at the pinnacle event. The athlete may have their support withdrawn. Coaches may have their employment terminated. The sports themselves may have their funding reduced or even withdrawn entirely.

Oddly enough the same readiness to impose consequences is not displayed by the machinery of sporting administrative bodies when it comes to holding themselves accountable to performance outputs. With perhaps one notable exception, national institute organisations will rarely exercise the same standards when it comes to employed support staff who are assigned to the respective sports.

Of course, national sporting federations will also not generally apply the same level of scrutiny when it comes to the accountability of their own management and administrative staff. This phenomenon might be described as the 'turkeys don't vote for Christmas' scenario.

ACCOUNTABLE TO WHOM?

In professional sports, holding each player in the process accountable is somewhat more straightforward given that each member of support staff is recruited and employed by the same organisation. When 'high performance' support is provided by an agency that is external to the sport, there are inevitably issues of ownership and accountability.

The situation whereby service providers are employed by another organisation is common with many individual and Olympic sports in various parts of the world. To some extent this is a consequence of the fact that these sports do not boast the resources of professional teams. Another factor is the way funding for these sports is allocated by government agencies.

In some instances, this means that the coach or whoever is ostensibly leading the 'high performance unit' is bound by constraints whereby the only funded support available is via the national or regional institute system. Clearly this can be a major obstacle, given that the providers involved ultimately serve a different master.

If members of the support team are not directly employed and therefore accountable to the sport then clearly it becomes more difficult to ensure that everybody is working towards the same goal and bound by their contribution to these outcomes.

Fatally, in some national 'high performance' systems there can even be a situation whereby there are essentially no consequences when ultimately providers fail in their duty to serve the sport.

A CAUTIONARY TALE...

This story comes from a Winter Olympic sport. The men's and women's national teams were considered a high probability for winning multiple gold medals, based on the history of every previous major championships to date, as well as recent performances. The fact that this was a niche event in which the nation had unmatched history, and few other nations contested the event seriously, was also helpful.

For these very reasons, every branch of athlete support was thrown at the programme by the institute of sport, regardless of need. For the most part this provision was unwarranted and certainly not requested. This is a skill sport in which performance is not bound by physiology, or indeed reliant on generic athletic qualities (strength, power, or speed). Hence, the involvement of the miscellaneous support staff was largely motivated by the lure of the reflected glory afforded by association with a gold medal-winning programme.

When the Winter Olympics came round the men's and women's teams not only failed to win gold, but came away with zero medals. This was unprecedented in their history.

In the debrief that followed, athletes and coaches identified the misguided and inappropriate involvement of miscellaneous support providers and associated distractions as major factors which adversely affected their preparation and performance in the event.

Despite these damning findings, those involved were not sanctioned or effectively held to account in any way. Indeed, one of the service providers who was most culpable was promoted to a senior role in the national institute of sport organisation not long afterwards.

NO COMPETING AGENDAS

Most commonly issues occur when the key performance indicators that each discipline or team member is held accountable to takes little or no account of what is best for the athlete and coach in relation to the ultimate performance goals.

In his treatise on the management and success of a high performance unit, Phil Coles warns against a situation where respective disciplines are working in isolation from each other.

"An integrated approach of the HPU to improve each player's athletic capability means the unit as a whole may then be held accountable for any success or failure"

— Phil Coles

Once more, this scenario is more difficult to achieve when service provision is delivered by an external agency. One of the most frequent criticisms of the institute of sport model is that the respective disciplines operate as silos. The worst case is that providers representing the respective disciplines not only work in isolation, but the disciplines themselves operate in competition with each other.

An associated problem arises from each respective area of athlete support essentially striving to justify their own existence. Representatives of the respective disciplines are therefore driven to promote their own area of service provision, with little regard for any identified need from the sport. In this instance, service providers are judged by what traction and involvement they gain with the sport or athlete, regardless of whether this involvement is warranted.

Here we see there is the potential for competing agendas is considerable. Where service providers are motivated by, and held accountable to, interests other than those of the sport and the ultimate performance goals, clearly this cannot be considered 'high performance'.

IN CLOSING...

So, whilst the label 'high performance' is freely applied in different sports and organisations around the world, actually achieving a system of athlete support and a 'high performance unit' that merits the title is far more involved than it appears.

As we have explored in this chapter there are a number of obstacles that must be overcome. Whilst systems are evolving, the majority of sports and organisations around the world are still grappling with these issues. Given the size and complexity of the challenges involved, resolving this will be no easy task and there is some work to go until many sports and systems ascend to true 'high performance'.

The Rise of the Movement Specialist

P ractitioners and coaches working in the field of performance sport will have noticed the emergence of a new job description in recent times. A casual search on sites such as LinkedIn will reveal a burgeoning number of people describing themselves as a 'movement specialist', 'movement coach', or some variation thereof. In this chapter we will explore these developments and attempt to explain this phenomenon.

FILLING THE VOID...

Few could argue with the message that there is a need to better understand athletic movement, as well as the processes by which these capabilities are acquired and expressed in competition. The growth of the movement specialist field is also indicative of a niche, and suggests that perhaps this is a need that is currently not being adequately addressed, even in the realms of elite and professional sport.

During early conversations with pioneers of the movement skill coaching 'movement' I applauded them for bringing the spotlight onto movement skills coaching; however, I did suggest that surely what they describe as a 'movement specialist' is simply a practitioner (or sports coach) who has an eye for movement and pays proper attention. Whilst there was an admission that this should be true, their response was that what they had repeatedly observed in professional sport was that this role was typically not being fulfilled by the support staff or coaching team in many instances. More specifically, too often the weights room strength coach, the positional coach, or indeed the athletic trainers on staff do not provide the necessary attention or expertise in this area.

On reflection I had to concede on this point. For instance, track and field athletics is a sport that exemplifies the critical importance of attention to detail with respect to movement execution, and technical development is an integral part of athletics coaching and the training undertaken in the sport. Indeed one of the key messages in presentations I have given for this audience is that physical preparation is so integral to technical development and ultimately performance in track and field that it must be undertaken by a practitioner who possesses a complete understanding of not only athletic movement in general, but also the event and the specifics of the technical model for each athlete.

DEVELOPING ATHLETIC SKILLS...

Turning our attention to developing performance in other sports (notably team sports), recent studies also highlight the importance of specific training to develop the particular motor abilities that underpins the performance attribute. For instance, studies investigating speed development identify that the most effective of the training modes employed to develop speed qualities was the specific training for the movement itself - i.e. sprinting. This has clear implications for practitioners who work in these sports. The value of movement skill training has likewise been demonstrated as an integral component of successful 'injury prevention' and rehabilitation regimens.

These findings beg the question how well equipped are the strength and conditioning specialists and physiotherapists who are most often charged with delivering the specific movement skill training in a performance or a rehabilitation context. If the practitioner is lacking the requisite skills and expertise in this area then clearly this is a major issue that will adversely affect the athletic development of the athletes concerned.

EYE FOR MOVEMENT...

The areas of injury prevention and rehabilitation also illustrate this point quite clearly. The effectiveness of screening for injury risk is entirely dependent upon the ability of the observer to detect and correctly interpret any aberrant movement patterns demonstrated by the athlete. Moreover, as 'live' screening in a real sports context is arguably the most illuminating, the practitioner should ideally be able to observe and interpret the movement behaviours demonstrated by the athlete in their training or practice environment.

Clearly this requires a very highly developed 'eye' for movement, in combination with an awareness and understanding of the sporting context. This is not something that is typically provided for in the standard education and practical training of practitioners who work in the area of sports injury.

Movement skills instruction and associated training is an integral aspect of injury prevention interventions that are shown to be effective in reducing injury. Once more this does have implications for those who design and deliver this training in the field. Do those involved possess the knowledge and expertise to adequately provide the quality of coaching and feedback required to elicit improvements in the movement skills involved (jumping, landing, specific changing direction manoeuvres)?

A final example comes from the management and rehabilitation of running injuries. A number of studies and authorities in the field point to the fact that the most potent interventions involve some manner of gait retraining. Clearly this implies that the practitioners responsible for treatment and rehabilitation must possess a detailed knowledge and deep understanding of running mechanics, and the ability to effect the necessary coaching intervention to retrain running gait patterns observed in previously injured running athletes. Once more, these are areas in which many practitioners working in sport at all levels are likely to be found lacking.

MOVING FORWARDS...

The rise of the movement specialist indicates, albeit indirectly, that there is a greater need for specific knowledge of kinesiology and specialist expertise in athletic movement. Such a need has been demonstrated in the numerous instances described in this chapter, in the contexts of both sports performance and sports injury.

So perhaps there is a call for movement specialists. That said, a great deal of work is required in order to avoid this becoming a nebulous term. We need to define what constitutes a 'movement specialist'. We must stipulate the competencies involved. Finally we need to find a way that this can be independently assessed in order for this title to be meaningful, rather than being self-ordained, as is currently the case.

More generally, there is certainly a need for greater recognition and awareness of these critical gaps in practitioners' knowledge, understanding, and expertise. These areas should be provided for in the preliminary education and ongoing training of practitioners who wish to specialise in sports performance and sports injury.

Ultimately, there is no short cut to developing our understanding and eye for movement. It will be up to the practitioner to hold themselves accountable, and take individual responsibility for investing the necessary time to observe and understand athletic movement in general, as well as the specifics and nuances of the sport(s) they are involved with. As practitioners in sport we should all be movement specialists.

Section Three – Principles

What Do We Mean by 'Athletic'? Pillars of Athleticism

Practitioners working in the realms of physical preparation, 'strength and conditioning', athletic development, sports coaching and sports medicine all share the desire that their athletes become more 'athletic'. Feats of athleticism can be readily recognised and appreciated. Yet observers and practitioners alike would struggle to describe with any clarity or detail what exactly constitutes 'athleticism'. Clearly we must first define qualities such as athleticism in order to understand how we might go about developing them. From a talent identification and talent development viewpoint, what do we need to identify and develop in a young athlete? In this chapter we aim to elucidate what athleticism is, and explore the constituent parts that underpin athleticism.

ATHLETICSM IS MULTIFACETED...

There are many facets of athleticism. These various capacities and capabilities span and cross-over between the sensory, perceptual, motor control, and neuromuscular realms. Each of these components we will introduce in turn, and describe in detail how they underpin athleticism.

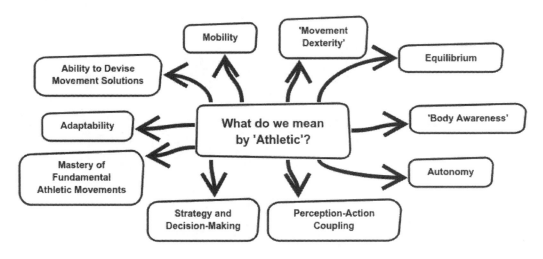

Figure 4: What do we mean by 'Athletic'?

1.   Mobility
Clearly if the athlete's ability to achieve certain positions and ranges of motion is restricted or constrained by a lack of mobility this is not conducive to athleticism. An important distinction needs to be made here between mobility and flexibility. Mobility constitutes a blend of flexibility, strength and stability. Flexibility training is generally complementary to mobility; however, mobility is active, whereas flexibility is broadly passive. Mobility comprises the ability to move through ranges of motion in a dynamic

fashion (often weight-bearing). Moreover, mobility demands that the athlete possesses the strength and functional capacities to maintain stability and postural integrity as they actively move through these ranges of motion.

2. Body Awareness

Practitioners often speak about athletes being 'body aware'. In this context, body awareness pertains to the degree and accuracy of the athlete's perception of position, orientation and sensation in relation to their body and limbs. This mind-body connection is rarely spoken about in the sporting realm, despite the importance of sensorimotor aspects in relation to motor control and coordination. The athlete's 'feel' for their own body and its interaction with the environment during a particular movement involves integrating a range of somatosensory input. The acuity of an athlete's perception in this regard tends to be quite specific to position and orientation in 3-dimensional space. For instance, an athlete might demonstrate good body awareness when standing upright and facing forwards with eyes open, but this is not necessarily be the case when placed in a less familiar position or orientation – for example, when hanging upside down. Developing 'global' body awareness ultimately requires the athlete to be exposed to a range of different postures, orientations, and movements in order to grow familiar with them and develop their acuity of perception in different contexts. For these reasons, gymnastics is a great tool for developing body awareness in a more global way. Specifically, the athlete is exposed to a variety of positions and postures, moving through different planes and axes of motion (rolling, rotating etc), and body orientations.

3. Equilibrium

I choose the term 'equilibrium' over 'balance' for a number of reasons. The first is that there are a variety of components to balance (static balance, dynamic balance, dynamic stabilisation). Furthermore each of these respective balance components involve weight-bearing in an upright posture. Equilibrium on the other hand encompasses not only the different components of balance in a weight-bearing stance, but also includes non-weight-bearing activities. For instance, equilibrium equally applies to the maintenance of posture and buoyancy in the water when swimming. Equilibrium also comprises body control in 3-dimensional space when moving through the air - for example when jumping, running, swinging, tumbling etc. Body awareness in different orientations as described previously is therefore a foundation quality.

4. Movement Dexterity

Dexterity concerns a high degree of coordination in movement, and as such is generally considered in the context of 'fine' motor skills. Dexterity encompasses aspects such as precision, 'touch' or 'feel', timing, and rhythm. Dexterity is most often spoken about in relation to the hand (manual dexterity). However, dexterity also relates to the remaining limbs and limb segments, for instance the lower limb when we are speaking about locomotion, and the concept of lower limb dexterity has recently been proposed [28].

Movement dexterity therefore pertains to all movement skills, whether global athletic movements or sports skills. Once again, possessing movement dexterity relates to precision, touch/feel, timing and rhythm when performing these various movement tasks. Movement dexterity thus comprises a host of somatosensory and sensorimotor qualities, which is far beyond what is normally considered with respect to neuromuscular control and coordination. Furthermore, these qualities and capabilities underpinning dexterity are demonstrated during both familiar and novel tasks.

5.   Mastery of Fundamental Athletic Movements

Elite performers clearly demonstrate mastery of the motor skills in their sport. In addition to these specific sports skills, a number of fundamental athletic movement skills can be identified that are common across sports. These include gait/locomotion, jump/land, lift, squat, lunge, balance, throw, catch, push, pull, twist/rotate, and pivot. Regardless of the sport, possessing true athleticism implies that the athlete exhibits mastery of these 'common' athletic movements. Even at elite level the degree of mastery of fundamental athletic movement skills cannot be assumed. This is particularly the case in complex sports with a significant tactical element, and among those who have lacked a comprehensive programme of physical preparation during their development years. The declining levels of fundamental movement skills among children has been highlighted previously; as such, this is likely to become an increasingly prevalent issue across sports, even among those who attain elite level.

6.   Autonomy

Perhaps the most abstract of the pillars we have encountered so far, but athleticism requires that the athlete is able to operate autonomously. For an athlete to demonstrate true athleticism, they cannot be dependent upon external feedback or instruction to properly execute a task. An athlete must therefore develop the ability to utilise 'intrinsic' feedback derived from the task and their own sensation and perception in order to execute athletic movements. The quality of intrinsic feedback comprises elements such as body awareness that we have spoken about before. By extension, the capacity to self-correct involves the ability to 'review' and utilise this intrinsic feedback to (independently) refine movement skill execution between repetitions. This feedback loop and ongoing correction and refinement occurs both in training and in a competition environment. Practitioners must remain aware of this when coaching athletes; the aim is to develop autonomy, not to foster dependency.

7.   Adaptability

The ability to adapt to different conditions is clearly important. The athlete must be able to execute athletic skills in different environments, and to adapt their movement skill execution to the environmental conditions faced at any given time. Once again this comprises the ability to utilise intrinsic feedback to modulate skill execution both within and between repetitions. However it also involves 'higher order' cognitive function - for instance, judging and evaluating the task environment in order to tailor skill execution to the conditions faced. Developing adaptive athletic skills once again comes back to coaching and the learning environment in which skills are developed. As we have spoken about, the nature of coaching input can be a critical factor. Likewise, the timing and frequency of the provision of external feedback are also relevant considerations.

8.   The Ability to Devise Movement Solutions

On an elemental level, an athlete's 'movement behaviour' in a training or competition environment can be conceptualised as a problem-solving process. In essence the athlete must devise satisfactory movement solutions for the given task encountered. The first step for devising these movement solutions involves perceiving the 'action opportunities' afforded by the task. These action opportunities, or 'affordances' for action, must also be evaluated in the context of the particular constraints associated with the task, such as the rules of the game or stipulations made by the coach, so this will narrow the range of options available. The range of movement solution the athlete has at his or her disposal will also depend on the size of their body and length of their limbs. Athletes therefore perceive their environment and the movement task within that environment in a way that is scaled to their body and limb lengths. Finally, the options available to the athlete will be based on their perception of their own capabilities or 'effectivities'. A virtuoso athlete who demonstrates extraordinary athleticism may therefore be able to come up with movement solutions that are not available to other mortals.

9.   Perception-Action Coupling

Up until now the discussion of athleticism has encompassed 'closed skill sports' for which the task and environment are relatively unchanging, and timing of the performance of the movement skill is largely predictable and predetermined (examples include fixed target shooting, and the field events in athletics). However, for a large number of sports the execution of athletic movement skills occurs in response to a stimulus, so that perception (stimulus) and action (athletic movement) are coupled. This might be a simple reaction task - for example, reacting to the gun in a sprint event. In other sports, the process of perception-action coupling can be far more complex as the athlete must perceive and respond to a range of cues, and a task environment that might be constantly changing. Demonstrating athleticism in these sports therefore demands additional sensory-perceptual aspects underpinning the successful coupling of perception and action.

10. Strategy and Decision-Making

Expressing athleticism in complex sports is incumbent upon a host of sensory-perceptual abilities to devise task solutions in real-time, and determine when to initiate an appropriate movement response. Using the example of an evasion sport, moment by moment the athlete must come up with a movement strategy as they go, and often then adapt in response to changing external factors and other players in the task environment. This encompasses not only perceiving a changing environment and constantly evaluating 'action opportunities', but also making decisions on when to act, when not to act, and which of the movement options available at that particular instant is most appropriate.

IN SUMMARY...

So, there we have it: rather than comprising any one single quality, athleticism comprises a host of different elements. In discussing each of the respective pillars of athleticism we have identified, it becomes evident that a number of the respective aspects are interconnected and many share elements in common. Identifying and developing the qualities that underpin athleticism is arguably relevant to all practitioners. After all, the benefits of possessing athleticism are widely recognised at all levels of competition; and this transcends across all sports disciplines. Identifying the pillars of athleticism marks an important first step on the path. Clearly the next step is to elucidate how we develop each of the constituent parts in order to improve athleticism. But that is a topic for another day.

The Training System Trap

Within the realms of training, coaching and even sports medicine there is often pressure to align with a particular 'training system' of regimented way of working. The urge to belong to one camp or other is common and beguiling. Proponents for the latest in vogue training system are often vocal and active in pursuing new recruits. It is also not uncommon to see much haranguing of those who subscribe to alternative approaches or competing training systems. In this chapter, we delve deeper into this notion of ready-made 'operating systems'. For instance, are there potential down-sides to adopting a training system? We will also explore an alternative path of being systematic in our approach, versus 'having a system'.

'YOU MUST HAVE A SYSTEM'...

Young practitioners especially are seduced by the idea of adopting a ready-made training system. There is security in following a system or structure that is recognised and popular in the field. Even when the details of the methodology of the 'system' are not well defined, being able to say I practice *insert name*'s system is perceived to reflect back on the practitioner in a way that lends them credibility.

Equally experienced coaches and practitioners are likewise not immune from this urge to ally themselves to a system of practice. Being part of a tribe lends the practitioner a feeling of safety and security. As we will speak about later in the chapter, time and experience often only serves to strengthen the bond with the chosen system.

> "People can maintain an unshakeable faith in any proposition, however absurd, when sustained by a community of like-minded believers"
>
> – Daniel Kahneman[25]

On the other side of the compulsion to commit to a system, those who wish to remain a 'free agent' are also often made to feel quite uncomfortable. This can be a little bit like organised religion. Those who choose their own path must guiltily admit to not following a recognised system, and often face scorn for doing so.

SHORTCOMINGS OF ANY SYSTEM

Even the best training system cannot be expected to fit all individuals. As such, even if you had a hypothetical system that is effective for 80% of all athletes, inevitably this system will fail to meet the needs of 1 in 5 athletes you come across.

Some coaches and practitioners recognise this and are happy to accept these odds. Others simply choose not to entertain this idea at all and place the blame on the athlete for not complying well enough.

IT'S A TRAP!

In the title of this chapter we used the term training system 'trap'. Taking the step to ally to a particular system inevitably tends to restrict practice. However, the removal of freedom also rids the practitioner of troubling feelings of uncertainty.

When you accept a system as your personal saviour there is no longer any need to explore the unknown and navigate uncharted waters; this is part of the appeal.

Adopting a system in turn often leads to 'confirmation bias'. Having chosen to ally oneself to a way of operating it is natural to then seek out evidence which is supportive of the path chosen. By extension, there is an urge to either disregard or dismiss anything that conflicts with the chosen way.

In addition to being selective when it comes to sourcing and interpreting 'evidence', confirmation bias also extends to the tendency to gravitate towards others who share the same viewpoint. All of this serves to deepen the conviction in the chosen system. The practitioner's position thereby becomes more entrenched over time.

The urge to cling to a system for the feelings of certainty and security this offers is understandable. Equally it is a security blanket that has a price. Being shackled to a training system not only restricts practice but can also distort perception. In particular, it does tend to constrain the ability to think critically. After all, critical thinking is reliant on a readiness entertain alternative explanations and different perspectives.

BEING SYSTEMATIC VERSUS 'HAVING A SYSTEM'...

So, we have established that any training system has shortcomings, and at best the chosen system will only be a good fit for a certain proportion of the athletes you will encounter. We have also made the case that being a devotee of any system is to be avoided in the interests of freedom and critical thought. Does this mean the answer is to reject the idea of a system entirely and simply freestyle?

Well, as usual, it is a little more involved than that.

Directing the training process to achieve certain outcomes requires the practitioner to be methodical and coherent in their approach. Shotgun programming that lurches in one direction then another clearly has very little coherence and is unlikely to bring the desired outcomes, particularly over an extended timeline.

So whilst pledging allegiance to a single system to the exclusion of all others is to be avoided, there remains a need to be systematic.

PRINCIPLES ARE FOUNDATIONAL...

"Principles are few. The man who grasps principles can successfully select his own methods. The man who tries methods, ignoring principles, is sure to have trouble."

— Ralph Waldo Emerson

As we have spoken about no single training 'system' is appropriate and successful with all individuals. Just as no training system is all good, the odds are it is not all bad either. Whilst the particular method or approach might not fit for all purposes and all individuals, equally there will be instances and individuals where it is suitable.

If we are clear on governing principles this allows freedom to select methods from a variety of sources and modify accordingly. Whilst this might be sacrilegious to purists and devotees of a particular system, it is possible to take the best parts without committing to any one camp.

ATHLETE 'ARCHETYPES'...

In a given sport or athletic event there are a range of athlete 'archetypes' that the coach or practitioner will commonly encounter. A certain archetype will suit a particular technical model. An example of this is track and field athletics would be a 'speed-jumper' versus a 'power-jumper'.

Likewise, there are archetypes that respond to very different approaches to training. An example of this might be a 'work horse' who craves and responds to high training volume, versus a 'Thoroughbred' who does best with quite brief high output sessions and requires extended regeneration in between.

Whilst the notion of athlete archetypes is useful, it is important to recognise that in reality this is a spectrum. On that basis, rather than assigning athletes to a pigeon hole, it is more of a judgement of where each athlete sits on that continuum between the opposite extremes or 'poles' of athlete archetypes.

ADAPTABLE 'TEMPLATES'...

With these caveats in mind, over time and experience working with a variety of athletes in different sports a practitioner will nevertheless evolve 'templates' of working with different athlete archetypes. Having acquired this experience, the practitioner is then able to select from these templates, whilst understanding the need to adapt them to suit the purpose and individual.

As we have spoken about, it is most useful to think in terms of a continuum of archetypes, rather than discrete categories. Moreover, individual athletes also vary widely where they are on their journey. The athlete's background and training history must be considered, as this will inevitably leave traces, which in turn impact how they deal with and respond to the training prescribed.

Conversely, novice athletes might be raw but they also bring less baggage, with respect to movement behaviour and preconceptions. Having a blank canvass makes a coach's job more straightforward. There are also more easy wins at this stage. In contrast, re-education and breaking movement habits inevitably requires more time and effort on part of both coach and athlete.

INDIVIDUALISED DELIVERY...

As we have alluded to, athletes vary in their response to the training prescribed. For a given type of training, at one end of the spectrum there are 'super-responders', in the middle ground you find 'responders' to varying degrees, and at the other extreme 'non-responders'. It follows that the manner and rate of progression when programming and delivering training must also be individual.

Individualisation also often comes down to the detail of adapting the plan and manipulating sessions each day. Essentially, this is the only way to be responsive to the myriad of different factors at play when dealing with biological systems and athletes who are subject to a host of variable influences and stressors outside the training and competition environment.

Individualised delivery also concerns how the plan is presented, and the manner of training delivery day to day. For many, a good approach is 'fail quickly, fail better... ultimately succeed'. In contrast, a perfectionist athlete will be very uncomfortable with this, and may quickly become despondent and shut down when faced with this approach. Whilst this may be an area of personal development for this athlete archetype, in the short term there will be a need to devise sessions to ensure a high probability of small and regular wins.

IN CLOSING: BE LIKE WATER...

By definition, it seems highly improbable that there will be a training system that is optimal for all individuals, or even applicable at all times for the same individual.

Resisting the urge to belong to any one camp or training system helps avoid becoming entrenched and the myopic view of the world that comes from this position. Whilst this freedom and uncertainty may be uncomfortable for some, it does allow you to retain the independence to evaluate without bias and to think critically.

Moreover, 'going rogue' allows the freedom to pick and choose. Having a clear understanding of governing principles also allows blending elements from a variety of systems. Hereby we adopt an adaptive approach to meet the needs of the individual and the situation at hand.

So discard the security blanket. Cast off the shackles that come with being bound to a regimented system of operating. Freedom permits exploration and allows practice to evolve over time. It is possible to be systematic without being a slave to a training system.

To paraphrase Bruce Lee, 'be like water'. Fit your approach to the individual; be responsive and adaptable, but nevertheless remain clear on the direction the current is flowing, the ultimate destination, and the general course that will take you there.

Specificity and the Simulation Trap

A recurring topic raised during discussions with young coaches particularly is the notion of 'sport-specific' programming. Specificity is much misunderstood, or at best incompletely understood, in relation to training prescription and programming. Our task is to prepare the athlete for the rigours of training and competing. Nonetheless, rather than attempting to train the sport into the individual, we should train the individual in the sport. In this sense the sport (or sports) provides the context, but the focus remains tailoring physical preparation and athletic development to the individual. This is a subtle but important distinction as we will explore in this chapter.

PRINCIPLES OF SPECIFICITY...

The notion of specificity is fundamental to the training process, as encapsulated in the acronym 'SAID' - i.e. specific adaptation to imposed demands. As I wrote about a number of years ago, there are various implications and applications of specificity in relation to training adaptation [29].

It is easy to see how the simulation trap arises. The more similar the training stimulus to the outcome measure the greater the immediate transfer is likely to be. It would appear to follow that if training prescribed replicates the sport then this will provide the best transfer to performance.

FLAWS IN APPLICATION...

Whilst on the surface this appears sound in theory, this short term and simplistic view of transfer of training effects is ultimately flawed. Highly movement specific training modes can be considered 'transfer training'. Such training modes inherently do not lend themselves to a high degree of force application - hence the degree of mechanical and morphological adaptation is very limited.

Fundamentally, a prerequisite for 'transfer training' is that the preceding training cycles have provided the foundation adaptation and increases in capacity, so that there is actually something to transfer.

By extension, a large part of the preparation undertaken by athletes will comprise training modes that appear quite generic. For instance, in the case of strength and power development, the requisite mechanical and morphological adaptation is often best provided by conventional heavy resistance training modes. Whilst these training modes might at first glance be dismissed as generic or 'non-specific', they nevertheless serve an important function in the physical preparation of athletes in a range of sports.

FUNCTIONALITY AND CONTEXT...

Moving beyond the realms of strength and power development, in all sports there are numerous other instances of training interventions employed to build capacity or capability, which would not be readily considered sport-specific. Examples include metabolic conditioning regimens designed to develop a specific quality (aerobic capacity, anaerobic capacity, anaerobic speed reserve), which on the surface bear very little resemblance to the athlete's chosen sport or athletic event.

Once again, these training interventions fulfil an identified need, and develop the athlete's capacity or capability to perform. Yet they do not simulate or replicate the sport of athletic event.

> "All functionality is context dependent, so that one has to examine every exercise in terms of the neuromuscular and metabolic functions that it is intended to improve"
>
> — Mel Siff

TERMINOLOGY...

Certain authorities in the field have attempted to reconcile these issues by introducing the term 'biomechanically relevant' in preference to 'sport-specific'. Regardless of which of these terms is employed, any narrow definition of specificity (or relevance) that is bound to 'dynamic correspondence' ultimately fails to consider a number of wider implications.

As stated earlier, our task is to prepare the athlete for the rigours of training and competing in their sport. For a given sport there is a characteristic extrinsic risk profile – essentially the potential areas for dysfunction and common injuries that arise from participating in that sport over time.

One important aspect of physical preparation therefore is putting countermeasures in place to address or counteract the repetitive stresses and predominant movements that are characteristic of (or specific to) the particular sport. These countermeasures are likely to involve exercises that are the biomechanically opposite to the actions involved in the sport.

EDUCATING OUR AUDIENCE...

Given how pervasive the concept of 'sport specific training' has been, once we have found clarity ourselves, there remains a need to educate coaches, athletes and even parents on this topic.

To illustrate this point, a couple of years ago I became involved in training three national-level swimmers. One important outcome the coach wanted was an improvement in their race starts. To that end, I employed relevant dry land training as well as spending time on pool deck providing specific coaching and instruction on starting from blocks and from the wall.

However, the coach was much less happy with the dry land training I prescribed in the weights room. Essentially, the reaction was one of outrage that the strength training modes for the upper limb particularly were not replicating the swim stroke, as he had expected. I explained my rationale – I took him through each of the exercises prescribed and explained their purpose, and my intention to develop and restore function at the shoulder girdle in particular.

In this way the physical preparation was ultimately supporting the swimmers ability to train consistently in the pool. The exercises prescribed, whilst on the surface appearing 'non-specific, were indirectly serving performance goals by guarding against the overuse injuries that are common in the sport.

In this case, the training prescribed was appropriate – and specific to – the desired outcome. Yet the dynamic correspondence between training and sporting activity was essentially zero – the training modes clearly did not simulate or replicate the movement in the sport. As stated previously, necessarily the countermeasures employed in training were by definition quite opposite and contrary to the sporting activity.

A WIDER VIEW...

These discussions, and the case study presented, exemplify the need for a wider and more considered view of what specificity means, in relation to the needs of the athlete, and in the context of the sport(s) in which they participate. In a previous chapter we spoke about the paradoxical relationship between simplicity and complexity in training. Once again, a simplistic view of specificity as simulation is at odds with the nuances and complexities of physical preparation and athletic development.

Conversely, taking a wider and longer-term view in relation to transfer of training effects allows us to consider how different methods can have application for building capacity and capability. Dynamic correspondence will then come into play with the transfer training modes we subsequently employ to build upon these foundations and take advantage of the residual training effects to facilitate the expression of the qualities developed in the context of the sport.

Section Four – Process

The Puzzle of Programming Training for Humans

The universal starting point when I engage in mentoring young practitioners is a 'SWOT analysis', to identify areas where they require development. A frequent response and common theme is the planning and programming of training. Before we get into the puzzles to solve when programming physical preparation, let us begin with a revelation: athletes are humans not machines. Input does not necessarily equal output. When working with athletes we must understand that we are dealing with inherently complex and highly dynamic biological systems. The task of designing a training plan for an athlete, or indeed a group of athletes, is therefore far from straightforward.

In this chapter we will unmask the flaws in the conventional wisdom that relates to planning and programming, including periodisation models. We will uncover the realities we face when programming training, explore the puzzles involved, and define the challenges we must resolve. Finally, we will outline a road map approach to guide planning physical preparation in a way that acknowledges the uncertainty, along with some strategies to help navigate the unknown and shifting terrain, to allow us to steer and adapt our course as we go.

FLAWS IN THE MODEL...

In a previous chapter, we discussed the training system 'trap'. Fundamentally, there are flaws in any model. The practice of adopting a single stereotyped approach, and applying it to all individuals and situations, is by definition inherently flawed.

> "Essentially, all models are wrong, but some are useful... "

> — George E.P. Box

ASSUMPTIONS VERSUS REALITY...

As identified by John Kiely [30], arguably the preeminent free-thinker on the topic, training systems and models for planning and periodisation rely upon a collection of shared assumptions. Any template or model by definition assumes that the response to training is (1) universal, (2) uniform, and (3) predictable. Whilst this textbook account of training adaptation presents a reassuring story for coaches and practitioners, it is nevertheless quite false.

The reality is that the response to training differs widely between individuals. Moreover, the training response is variable even within the same individual. Finally, training stress responses are influenced by a host of dynamic and interacting factors; all of which makes things inherently unpredictable.

Returning to the revelation we opened up the chapter with, humans do not respond in a stable or predictable manner whereby input equals output. Taking a machine approach to training humans is clearly inappropriate.

At face value, most would agree it is obvious that humans should not be treated as machines. Returning to John Kiely's writing, each athlete represents a 'complex adaptive system' [30]. Despite this, coaches and practitioners still commonly employ a spreadsheet approach to prescribing training. The notion that the athlete will be ready to lift 110% of their 1-RM on an arbitrary day or date simply because it was specified in advance as a 'very heavy day' on the programme is nonsensical. Nevertheless we see this approach practiced all the time.

PERCEPTION INFLUENCES TRAINING STRESS RESPONSE...

In his writing on the topic, John Kiely describes how perception is a powerful mediator of training stress responses that is overlooked by conventional models of training theory [24].

Essentially, how the athlete anticipates, perceives and therefore experiences the training stimulus has a profound effect on the training stress response. The critical element of perception shapes the responses that are elicited post training, even at a hormonal level. This affects the athlete's responsiveness to a training bout, and will also have implications for the athletes' readiness for subsequent sessions.

As Kiely identifies, a host of psycho-social factors can influence the perception and experience of training, and therefore the ensuing training stress response [24]. As such, there is far more to consider beyond simply manipulating conventional training variables, such as mode, frequency, intensity and volume.

PROGRAMMING CONUNDRUMS TO GRAPPLE WITH...

Challenge #1: Consistency/Monotony Paradox

There is a need for consistency in training input in order to elicit adaptation. Conversely, there is a need for variation, not least to guard against monotony. The difference between 'consistent' and 'monotonous' as it relates to the experience of training may to some extent come down to perception...

Challenge #2: Managing Perception

Understanding that perception of training is a powerful mediator of the response to the training stressor, how do we use this knowledge to manage how the athlete perceives and experiences training? Making the athlete clear on the purpose, and engaging them in the process, might permit more consistency in the training stimulus, whilst avoiding the negative aspects of training monotony.

Challenge #3: Diversity and Variability of Training Responses

Finally, the magnitude and time course of the response to training differs between individuals. These aspects also differ within the same individual, according to timing and previous exposure. How do we account for this when planning and programming training?

VARIETY WITH CONSISTENCY...

Relevant to both challenges #1 and #2, with a bit of guile and lateral thinking it is possible for the practitioner to provide variety within and between training cycles, whilst still providing a similar and congruent training stimulus.

For instance, incorporating variations and permutations of a training mode which are essentially equivalent can provide a superficial sense of variety or something different, whilst still basically working on the same elements. This is an example of accounting for perception in a way that supports effective training prescription and facilitates a more optimal experience of the training performed in order to enhance training readiness and responsiveness.

PILLARS OF PHYSICAL PREPARATION - THE 3 'C'S...

#Capacity - work capacity, horsepower, structural integrity

#Capability – Ability to control and coordinate each link of the kinetic chain during fundamental movements, adding degrees of freedom, and coping with additional neuromuscular challenge (an example would be overhead squat versus standard back squat)

#Correspondence – this encompasses 'transfer training modes' that favour short-term carryover; the weights room can also be rich for creating #context, in a way that facilitates motor learning, supporting skill acquisition, technical model

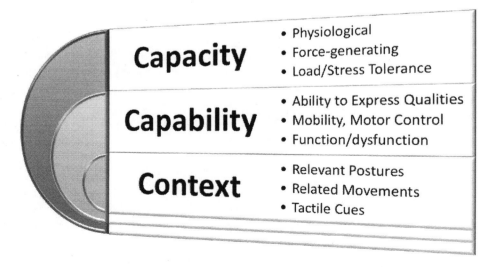

Figure 5: Capacity, Capability, Context

As we will explore in a later section, these same elements can be employed to devise a continuum of training modes.

A 'TAXONOMY' APPROACH TO ASSEMBLE THE TOOLBOX...

Taxonomy represents the process of classifying items or species in a systematic way. Famously, this approach has been used to create a hierarchical classification system to describe, categorise and organise all species of plants, animal and micro-organisms in the natural word.

The same approach can also be employed to create a classification system, and categorise training modes or menu items in an organised and coherent way, which can greatly assist planning and programming.

A practitioner can quickly populate their toolbox simply by coming up with different variations and permutations of common movements or training menu items, based upon certain task parameters.

Let us consider a squat. Load can be applied at various points on the athlete's body (e.g. front squat, back squat, overhead squat, hip belt squat etc. etc.). Various forms of load can be employed - for instance, barbell, dumbbell, kettle bell, cable, weighted vest. Stance can be varied, depth can be varied, tempo can be varied, ballistic variations (i.e. jump squat) can be employed. This example illustrates how you can quickly come up with a host of variations and permutations for a single movement, simply by manipulating a selection of task parameters in a systematic way.

ORGANISING THE TOOLBOX...

Returning to the three 'C's, we can use these elements (Capacity, Capability, and Context) to help sort and apply our new taxonomy of training modes. Capacity forms one pole, capability forms the middle part of the spectrum, and correspondence forms the opposite end of the continuum.

Training modes most geared to building capacity will sit at one end of the spectrum. Applying this to strength training, the variations that allow the most load to be handled and highest forces will comprise the 'capacity-building' end of the spectrum. Variations and progressions that develop capability will essentially form the middle portion of the continuum. At the other end of the spectrum will be coordination-oriented variations of the training mode that show the most resemblance or dynamic correspondence to the activity in the sport.

COHERENT INTEGRATION AND VARIATION...

Training variation is recognised as a critical component of successful training plans. As we have spoken about, variety is generally beneficial for maintaining engagement. Exposing the athlete to a greater array of training modes also helps create a wider movement playbook; hence a 'mixed methods' approach is particularly geared to developing capability. These benefits are apparent from a neuroplasticity viewpoint, and fostering what has been wonderfully termed the 'bliss of motor abundance' [31].

Equally, concerted application or exposure to a training stimulus is required to sustain adaptation, which is critical for building capacity in particular. Excessive variation or shotgun programming will fail to provide this consistency, and so will not allow for meaningful adaptation or increases in capacity.

It is important that there is some coherence in the manner in which variations and progressions of training modes are presented in the training plan. More specifically, it is important that the exercises in successive training cycles do not lurch from one end of the spectrum to the other.

Decisions on timing with respect to initiating progression should reflect the time course and degree of adaptation, which in turn is likely to vary between individuals. Clearly this will be very difficult to predict, and so is likely best managed in a responsive manner based upon ongoing observation and monitoring. Intensity can be manipulated (both up and down) on a day-to-day basis. Decisions on when to introduce new progressions of training modes will be made on a more periodic basis.

An example of this, which is sometimes observed in track and field athletics, is lurching straight from a concerted training block of heavy resistance training directly into a training cycle of plyometrics. From a coherence viewpoint, as well as taking best advantage of residual training effects and avoiding abrupt changes in the stimulus which might predispose to injury, it is important there is some step-wise progression in between.

VERTICAL AND HORIZONTAL INTEGRATION...

Vertical and horizontal integration refers to the coherent scheduling of different training components both within a training cycle (e.g. daily scheduling) and between training cycles.

The interaction between different elements within a day or training microcycle (e.g. training week or two-week cycle) is an important factor to consider. For instance, a particular session performed early in the day, or in the training week, will have residual effects that will affect the training sessions that are performed subsequently. The residual effect can be positive – such as a priming effect. Conversely, there are instances whereby the residual effect has an adverse effect, such as fatigue or soreness that impairs the athlete's ability to perform the training scheduled later in the day or the following day(s).

Residual effects also apply to successive training cycles. Preceding training cycles elicit delayed adaptations and progressive changes in capacity and capability that manifest themselves over time. In some instances these changes only become apparent some time after the cessation of the training block. A notable example is eccentric training, where there is often a considerable lag before positive changes become evident – usually weeks following the cessation of the eccentric training block.

Horizontal integration within the training macrocycle concerns this interaction between training components in successive training cycles. It is important when planning the training year to consider the associated residual and delayed effects. We must consider how we best manage and harness these effects.

MANAGING PERCEPTION OF TRAINING PRESCRIBED...

A major part of managing how the training is perceived by the athlete is to ensure they are clear on the 'why' for everything in the programme. It is unsafe to assume the purpose is obvious; we must make the effort to connect the dots so that the athlete has absolute clarity on the rationale and desired outcomes.

Similarly, relating each exercise or element of the programme to the athlete's sport or the specific demands they encounter in competition can be very powerful. Investing the time and making the effort to communicate this information - essentially presenting the case - can have a profound effect on how the athlete perceives the training prescribed.

Once the athlete has been part of the environment for a time, and attained a level of experience and understanding, it is important to allow the athlete some input on the programme. This will allow them to begin to feel it is a shared endeavour, rather than perceiving the programme as something that is dictated to them. Being more invested in the training plan positively impacts how the athlete perceives, experiences, and responds to the training they perform.

CONSIDERING DIVERSITY...

As noted in the previous section, the timing and rate of progression will differ between individuals. It follows that the way programmes are administered should include the facility to accommodate the time course of adaptation for individuals within the group.

All members of the group might begin the training year from approximately the same starting point and initial programme. Thereafter the practitioner administering the plan must allow for individual paths to deviate, based on how they respond. Essentially, the aim is that all members ultimately converge on the same end point at the culmination of the training year or macrocycle.

Practically, from experience athletes can be broadly grouped into archetypes, based upon where they sit on the 'responder' continuum and also how quickly they recover. This understanding of the athletes in the group may make the task of progressing training at different rates and time points more straightforward. That said, there will always be an ongoing need to monitor each individual's output and subjective measures of training stress, readiness and recovery.

MAP ORIGIN AND DESTINATION...

Devising a route begins with identifying (1) point of origin, and (2) the final destination. The first task for the practitioner therefore is to evaluate the starting position or entry point for each athlete. The next step is to define the desired end point, within the time-frame concerned (e.g. culmination of the training year or competition season).

Thereafter we must recognise that there are a number of potential routes between these two points. It is important to be adaptable in our planning and programming to allow for that.

Similarly, whatever route is chosen initially, it is possible to divert as the need arises to negotiate unforeseen issues, yet still continue to progress towards the desired final destination.

ADAPTING TO THE TERRAIN AND ADJUSTING COURSE...

> "Plans are of little importance but planning is essential"
>
> — Winston Churchill

The dynamic and unpredictable nature of training athletes calls for adaptable planning and responsive programming. We must of course establish start-point and map end-point in advance. However, whilst the practitioner might sketch out the steps in between ahead of time, practically the future is unknown and the path cannot be fully anticipated. With a final nod to John Kiely, we must recognise the topography and terrain are constantly changing. Practically, it would seem sensible therefore to restrict timelines when providing programmes in advance.

Critical components for adaptable planning and responsive programming include regular feedback and review mechanisms to inform and refine the ongoing process of training prescription. As mentioned previously, those athletes who possess sufficient understanding should also be afforded the opportunity to input on the ongoing programming process.

Yin and Yang of Preparation and Restoration for Injury Risk Management

A primary objective of the physical preparation performed by athletes is to confer some protection against the risk of injury. In this chapter I will make the case that there is a false separation in how we view training from a performance perspective versus injury prevention/rehabilitation. For the most part we are employing many of the same tools, or at least I contend we should be. The major difference is how the application of these tools is adapted to fit our purpose. In the sections that follow we will explore these issues. I will also make the case for greater integration and crossover, challenging as this may be to practitioners in their respective realms.

INJURY AND PERFORMANCE...

I opened this chapter with the contention that the separation between training in a performance context versus a sports injury context is somewhat spurious. If we reframe how we view performance and injury risk management we discover these elements are essentially inseparable; they are two sides of the same coin.

Performance outcomes and sports injury are inextricably linked. It has been demonstrated across a range of sports that injuries directly impact competitive success [32]. For instance, a study of the Champions League in professional soccer (the highest level of club competition in Europe) spanning over a decade showed the injuries sustained by a team was directly and negatively related to their progress [33]. In other words, teams suffering more injuries do not go as far in the competition. It has similarly been demonstrated that time loss injuries negatively impact team success in elite rugby union football [34].

To view this another way, if we are able to reduce the time lost due to injury via physical preparation we will have achieved an important performance outcome. A study of track and field athletes demonstrated that the major factor determining an athlete's success in achieving their goals was the extent to which they were able to avoid extended enforced breaks from their regular training due to illness or injury [35].

In other words, even if the only outcome of the athlete's physical preparation is that we help them to consistently participate in practice we are nevertheless delivering a critical performance outcome. We are literally providing the athlete the opportunity to succeed in their sport.

FAILINGS OF 'PREHAB'...

Too often 'prehab' simply consists of repurposed conventional rehabilitation exercises. Arguably these rehabilitation training modes are not optimal even within a rehabilitation setting, and they are certainly not appropriate for a healthy athlete.

A consistent theme identified in the injury prevention literature is the issue of compliance. The presumption among researchers and practitioners is that the solution is to better educate athletes and coaches on the purported benefits. The notion is that if the athletes and coaches only knew better they would become motivated to perform these interventions.

Perhaps we should consider that the issue might actually be the intervention itself. We should allow that the lack of motivation and compliance might in part be a reflection of the efficacy and appropriateness of the intervention, as opposed to the default position of assigning fault to the athlete and coach.

CONSIDERING MOTIVATION...

One of the major issue with retrofitting conventional rehabilitation exercises for use as 'prehab' with healthy athletes is that there is a stark difference in the level of inherent motivation in these two scenarios.

Clearly an injured athlete will be more receptive to essentially any intervention that is presented. Injured athletes are inherently motivated to try whatever might alleviate symptoms and help them return to competing. Understandably, pain and incapacity promote compliance; of course an athlete will continue to diligently perform the rehabilitation exercise as long as they perceive it has a chance of alleviating symptoms and helping to restore function.

By definition, an athlete who considers themselves to be healthy will of course not be so receptive to injury prevention interventions, or motivated to comply with these regimens over time. Rather, in this scenario, you motivate with challenge. Clearly if the athlete does not find the intervention challenging it is unlikely we will elicit motivation or compliance.

APPLICATION OF 'ADVANCED' TRAINING MODALITIES...

An extensive review demonstrated the application of strength training as a treatment and rehabilitation tool for musculoskeletal injury [36]. 'Mechano-therapy' is the term employed to describe the application of strength training modes to manage and rehabilitate injuries. Therapeutic applications heavy resistance training, eccentric training, isometric training are becoming more widely accepted, notably as a treatment modality for tendinopathy [37, 38].

The mechano-therapy conferred by the application of force via strength training and other 'advanced' training modes can have an analgesic component, termed 'mechanical hypoalgesia'. In essence, performing appropriate exercise can favourably modify pain responses and symptoms, and these effects can persist for hours at a time [38]. Strength training and other training modes can also elicit structural changes in 'mechano-responsive' tissues, including both contractile tissues (muscle) and connective tissues.

Advanced training modalities, when applied appropriately, therefore represent potent tools to increase capability and capacity in a way that improves function and confers protection by mitigating risk. These applications encompass both 'healthy' athletes and athletes with existing or prior injury [39].

GAPS IN THE TOOL KIT...

An expert consensus statement recommended that physicians working with sports teams should increase their knowledge of strength and conditioning principles and practice, as an integral part of their professional responsibilities [40]. I wrote a commentary making the wider case that a working knowledge of physical preparation process, including 'advanced training modalities, is a 'need to know' for all practitioners working in the field of sports injury [41].

Conversely, the practitioners who do possess experience and expertise in the physical preparation realm, i.e. the strength and conditioning staff, often lack the requisite detailed knowledge and depth of understanding in the field of sports injury. Once again, this points to a need for each member of the support staff to invest in continuing education and upskill in these respective areas.

DELIVERY MATTERS...

There are a number of issues of delivery that often adversely affect motivation and compliance with 'prehab' training. Preventive training is customarily the domain of the physiotherapist or sports medicine staff. By extension, these exercise are typically delivered in isolation from the athletes' physical preparation.

For instance, preventive training is often performed in a treatment setting or rehabilitation space, as opposed to the training facility where athletes perform their 'main' physical preparation. Even when preventive exercises are performed on the training pitch, such as the '11-plus' warm up and its derivations, typically this is administered in a way that is not readily associated with performance; and this is generally reflected in the level of engagement elicited among the athletes.

The issues of integration and physical space employed for delivery might appear minor, but this sends a message to the athlete that it is not important to their performance, but rather is merely ancillary training for the weak. Clearly this perception is compounded when the exercises employed are too conservative and not challenging. For an athlete who is presently not injured the sight of a thera band is not generally motivating.

RISK MANAGEMENT APPROACH...

Preventing injury is perhaps a lofty aim. However, if we establish known risks and identify what stresses the athlete is exposed to, we can prepare the athlete accordingly.

Physical and athletic preparation provide the means to implement countermeasures and manage the risks. A crucial aspect is that this preparation is delivered in the context of the sport and the performance model, rather than in isolation.

What constitutes acceptable risk is also dynamic. In particular, this will depend on the circumstances – for instance, where we are in the competition calendar, the relative importance of the event, and even where the athlete is in their career.

Ultimately the judgement on what constitutes 'acceptable risk' under the particular circumstances resides with the athlete and coach. The role of the practitioner is to inform this decision as far as possible. Once the decision is taken, the responsibility then switches to implementing strategies and countermeasures to best support the athlete in managing the risk.

BLURRED LINES…

There is often not a clear distinction between the realms of preventive training, therapeutic application of training injury management, and rehabilitation training. At the elite level particularly, at any given time even a 'healthy' athlete is likely to be managing some sort of niggle or pre-existing issue.

Another case where lines are necessarily blurred concerns the territorial boundaries for the respective practitioners concerned.

PROFILING RISK…

If we apply the model for sports injury developed in the literature [42], there are essentially three areas we need to explore in order to establish the risk profile for a given athlete.

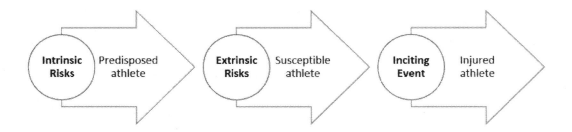

Figure 6: Causality of Sports Injury

The first element in the figure concerns the intrinsic risk profile of the athlete as an individual, based on known risk factors for injury, such as history of previous injury. The next step adds the extrinsic risks associated with the sport in which the athlete competes, including consideration of specific factors that relate to their individual role, game plan, or technical model. The final step involves examining the injuries that are prevalent in the sport, and delving into the mechanisms for the specific injuries observed, which would represent the 'inciting event' in the figure above.

In order to develop the plan we must establish the starting point for each individual. In other words, we need to define the intrinsic risk profile for each athlete. The first step is to undertake a thorough injury history. Relevant information will include training history, and prior exposure to coaching. This should be complemented with a comprehensive musculoskeletal assessment, including postural assessment, and a selection of validated clinical assessments of mobility and joint function.

We should also be vigilant for compensations and any apparent dysfunction. Inevitably there is a degree of subjectivity in assessing these aspects, albeit video recording can help to provide an objective record that we can use to independently verify our assessments. More importantly, we should conduct these assessments under live conditions, such as during performance testing, rather than the contrived and unrepresentative conditions more usually associated with 'functional screening' [43]. This evaluation should be complemented by actively observing the athlete during practice and competition to evaluate any mechanical factors that might predispose them to injury.

Extrinsic risks concern the environment in which the athlete operates. The specific constraints within which the athlete operates may differ according to their technical model or individual style, the tactical concerns (for instance, the playing style of the team), and the nuances of the playing position. The nature of the competition environment and associated extrinsic risk factors will also differ according to the venue and environmental conditions.

It can be illustrative to examine the common injuries for the sport and particular classes of athlete in the sport (such as different playing positions). Armed with this information, we can also take a deeper look at the mechanisms that are commonly observed for the particular injury identified within the sport.

FORENSIC APPROACH...

In the case of a 'healthy' (uninjured) athlete, we can seek to apply a 'prospective forensic approach' whereby we attempt to prevent the crime (injury) from happening in the first instance. In essence, we aim to anticipate the risks the athlete will be exposed to, and pre-emptively employ countermeasures to address the specific intrinsic risks established for the athlete.

When dealing with a previous or ongoing injury, this 'forensic approach' will obviously take a retrospective look. In this instance we are seeking to gather as much information as possible to establish how the injury occurred, and we might also infer likely causal factors.

Our analysis in this case should also extend to evaluating the residual effects and any compensations we can observe that are secondary to the injury. Once again, this information will be critical to informing what needs to be addressed to help mitigate the risk of a repeat occurrence.

DEFINING OBJECTIVES...

Clearly our aim from an injury risk management viewpoint is to take steps to mitigate the risks we have established for the sport and athlete.

An interesting discussion point is whether it is sufficient to return the athlete to baseline following injury. Clearly this is a challenge in itself. However, we must also take into account the fact that prior injury is the biggest known risk factor for future injury.

Since previous injury is now added to the athlete's risk profile, even if we successfully return athlete to baseline their risk for future injury is nevertheless still increased.

PRINCIPLES...

Borrowing from the pillars of physical preparation presented in the previous chapter, the principles that govern the injury risk management approach can be encapsulated with four 'C's. In addition to the three elements of **capacity**, **capability**, and **correspondence/context**, the presence of previous or ongoing injury adds a fourth: **cascade**.

Part of what **capacity** concerns in this context is increasing failure limits. Appropriate exposure to 'advanced' training modes, including heavy resistance training, offers the means to enhance structural integrity and to build stress tolerance. Developing extra capacity, in terms of physiological capacity, muscular strength, and strain capacity of non-contractile tissues, is protective. For instance, greater aerobic capacity renders the athlete more resilient and thereby better able to cope with fluctuations in acute training or competition workloads [44]. Likewise, better developed physical capacities appear to render some protection against injuries associated with high-speed running and sprinting [45].

From a **capability** viewpoint, part of the challenge when working with previous injury or ongoing symptoms is to find efficiencies, in order to reduce mechanical strain placed on the affected area.

Part of the genius of evolution is that the body has in-built 'redundancy'. In essence, reserve systems and extra functional capacity can be called upon to take the strain when a particular component is compromised or incapacitated. This reserve capability or 'functional redundancy' also extends to the motor system. Even when compromised by injury, we are able to draw upon what authors have described as 'the bliss of motor abundance' [31] to select one of a number of alternative motor strategies to achieve the movement objective. The adaptive motor strategies developed by an athlete when injured are however not necessarily optimal moving forward, and this may become a problem that needs to be solved further down the line.

Taking a more positive perspective, rehabilitation and injury management provides the motivation and the opportunity to make technical improvements to find a more mechanically efficient and more optimal way of doing things. In the presence of a pre-existing injury, an athlete no longer has the luxury of being sloppy in their practice and how they move. The experience of injury and the process that follows can hereby be advantageous from a capability and performance viewpoint, if the athlete is willing and able to full advantage of the opportunities afforded to become better.

As with any application of physical and athletic preparation, **context** is critical when approaching injury risk management. Practitioners working with healthy or injured athletes must invest the time to elucidate and consider the specifics of their performance model. For instance it will be necessary to identify mechanical factors, encompassing both kinetics (forces and torques) and kinematics (motion) at the level of each joint and the body as a whole.

When dealing with pre-existing injuries, or managing ongoing overuse injury, there is a need to consider and to address both cause and symptoms. Beyond this, there is also a need to consider the **cascade** of secondary factors and effects occurring subsequent the injury. This is encompassed within the 'what else, where else' principle that we will meet in the chapter that follows. Practically, we need to broaden the scope of the assessment, inspecting up and down the kinetic chain.

PILLARS OF PREPARATION AND RESTORATION...

There are three pillars of physical preparation from an injury risk management perspective:

- Strength training modalities,
- jump-land and plyometric training,
- and movement (re-) training.

Elements will often traverse disciplines and territories. It is particularly crucial that the physical and athletic preparation is undertaken in coordination with any ongoing treatment and manual therapy.

Combination general protection conferred by a comprehensive programme of physical preparation, supported by targeted application of specific training to address specific risk factors associated injuries identified prevalent sport or areas athlete prone.

APPROPRIATE CHALLENGE...

Returning to the different applications of preparation and restoration, as we have spoken about there is a need to cater to the respective needs of healthy athletes, versus symptomatic and injured athletes. Armed with our governing principles and a knowledge of the key pillars, appropriate challenge is the final piece that permits programme design and delivery to be geared to the respective audience.

With healthy athletes, you motivate with challenge. Working with the themes of capacity and capability there are a number of ways we can find to challenge the athlete. For instance, we can select training modes that target their weak links. There are similarly a host of options for challenging capability across the respective areas, particularly with respect to plyometrics and athletic movement skills. Harnessing the power of context can also aid engagement, by framing training modes in relation to the specifics of the athlete's performance model and competition scenarios.

Appropriate challenge is also central to delivery in both injury management and rehabilitation contexts. There will be a need to explore the boundaries of what the athlete can tolerate, and this will be guided by symptoms. However, within these constraints there is often considerably more scope than many practitioners realise. Pioneering practitioners in this space, notably in the extreme sports realms, have demonstrated what is possible with a willing athlete, even at relatively early stages in the rehabilitation process following major surgery such as ACL reconstruction.

Equally the boundaries with respect to what the athlete is able to tolerate will also be dynamic, fluctuating day-to-day, as well as progressing over time. With both chronic conditions and the rehabilitation process the time course for recovery varies, and the progression of symptoms and function over time does not trace a neat line. The practitioners involved must be alert to these changes and ready to modify the session on any given day. In turn, staged progression should be guided by achievement of benchmark criteria for capacity and capability, rather than working to arbitrary timeframes.

BRAVERY AND 'BUY IN'...

There is a common scenario of well-meaning practitioners essentially killing the athlete with kindness through excessive caution and overprotectiveness. Clearly an injured athlete has an air of vulnerability and the urge to wrap them up in cotton wool is understandable. Equally if we 'protect' the athlete from exposure to high forces and 'risky' activities during the injury management or rehabilitation process we will only render them more vulnerable to future injury.

If we accept that our task is to prepare the athlete to return to competition then we must progressively expose them to competition conditions and prepare them for the rigours involved during the rehabilitation and return to sport process. Clearly we do not want to impose demands that dramatically exceed their present capacity and capability to the extent we expose the athlete to undue risk of injury. Equally, there is a need to be brave. To best serve the athlete the practitioner we cannot indulge the urge to be conservative.

Of course the athlete needs to be brave and 'buy in' too. Inevitably there will be some apprehension involved, particularly in the early stages following injury. Taking a progressive approach to injury management and rehabilitation is entirely contingent upon the level of trust and consent from the athlete to engage with this process. Likewise, progression is ultimately dependent upon the athlete's willingness to attempt the next stage.

MANAGING MENTAL AND EMOTIONAL ASPECTS...

Psychological and emotional aspects represent important factors in the rehabilitation and injury management process. Perception is highly potent in this regard. For instance, both perceived stress and perceived recovery are reported to have a bearing on athletes' risk of suffering injury [46].

Fear and apprehension in relation to injury are somewhat self-fulfilling. Athletes who report being anxious about illness or injury prior to competition demonstrate a significantly higher likelihood of subsequently sustaining an injury [47]. We should acknowledge here that athletes' anxiety often related to symptoms. Equally, these data also point to the crucial role of the practitioner in helping to assuage the fears and anxieties of the athlete, particularly prior to and during major competition.

From an injury risk management perspective we must monitor and address psychological factors, particularly in those who have suffered an acute injury or are managing a chronic injury. Once again, apprehension is a perfectly natural response to injury. Equally we must help the athlete to overcome this as far as possible.

READINESS TO RETURN...

Anxiety and fear of (recurrent) injury should be recognised as a risk factor for those returning from injury. To mitigate this risk we must be vigilant and prepared to implement appropriate countermeasures to help the athlete to develop the necessary mental skills and coping strategies to reduce their anxiety in relation to re-injury. Psychological and emotional aspects should be included in the criteria for determining readiness to return to competition. Some psychometric tools to assess readiness to return to competition have been developed for this purpose [48].

There is also a particular need to address motor deficits observed post injury which persist for an extended period even once other metrics of strength and function have returned to normal range. These residual effects are evident in the altered biomechanics demonstrated by athletes, which may be observed under planned as well as reactive conditions.

Recent data indicate that the origin for these altered movement mechanics are both peripheral, due to disruption of mechanoreceptors at the joint and surrounding tissues, and central with neuroplastic changes at the level of the motor cortex and central nervous system. It appears that the disruption of sensory input is compensated for by adopting a 'visual-motor' control strategy that relies upon visual input to offset the loss of mechano-receptor input (sensory-motor strategy) [49].

Clearly these deficits in motor control will be exposed in the highly dynamic and unpredictable competition environment associated with team sports and racquet sports. The 'visual-motor strategy' might be adequate in a stable and predictable environment, but this becomes a problem when there is a need to visually scan and attend to motion of an implement, opponent(s), and team-mates. Adopting the risk management approach, these represent quite glaring issues that must be addressed to mitigate the risk of returning to sport.

An illustrative example is the recovery process following ACL reconstruction. The persisting high rate of adverse outcomes with this injury has led some authors to explore neuromuscular factors, as well as psychological readiness [50]. In particular, notable authors point to the need to consider neuroplasticity, and the need to retrain movement mechanics and the sensorimotor qualities that underpin them [51].

The process of re-learning and embedding movement skills will necessarily involve 'advanced' athletic skills. Once again, these investigations steer us into realms more commonly associated with athletic performance, including motor skill development. In particular, this will require practitioners who possess comprehensive knowledge and deep understanding of athletic movement, in order to guide the process of re-learning and refining these adaptive movement skills and associated capabilities.

Notable authors have recommended that late-stage rehabilitation and return to sport preparation should integrate 'neurocognitive' and 'visual-motor' approaches [51]. Progressions should therefore incorporate additional visual, perceptual, and motor skill tasks in order to challenge and restore sensorimotor capabilities. In this process we must account for the specific sensory-perceptual and cognitive aspects involved in perception-action coupling and decision-making elements in the sport. Practically the best way of achieving representative conditions to develop the appropriate qualities will involve a staged return to dynamic practice conditions with team-mates and opponents.

CRITERIA-BASED PROGRESSION AND DECISION-MAKING...

A critical implication of the psychological, emotional, and motor control aspects of 'readiness' is that we need to move away from timeframe-based rehabilitation and return to sport procedures.

Whatever the rationale for the time course chosen, this approach ultimately ignores the athlete. Recovery is nonlinear and highly individual. If we were to plot an athlete's recovery over time it would likely trace an erratic line with many fluctuations, rather than the tidy and predictable curve assumed by time-based protocols. Moreover, the host of psychological, sensorimotor, and motor skill aspects that govern readiness by definition defy arbitrary timelines.

IN CLOSING: TWO SIDES OF THE SAME COIN...

Performance outcomes and efforts to safeguard against injury are essentially inseparable. Adopting an 'injury risk management' perspective provides a framework that serves both of these aims. We need a more cohesive approach to the physical and athletic preparation undertaken for injury risk management. By necessity this new approach will transcend the traditional boundary lines between disciplines and their respective domains.

What are commonly considered 'advanced' training approaches in the physical preparation and athletic development domains represent necessary tools to safeguard the athlete and mitigate known risks associated with practice and competition in the particular sport. In particular, these approaches have important applications for managing injury and the rehabilitation process.

Finally, there is a need for a more individualised and responsive approach to return to sport, with progressions and decision-making on 'readiness' that is governed by criteria, rather than based on arbitrary timelines. Our approach to evaluation and preparation in this process will necessarily integrate physical, motor skill development, sensory-perceptual, and psychological elements.

Defining 'Performance Therapy'

What originally prompted the discussions on the theme of 'performance therapy' that feature in this chapter was a discourse that occurred on social media. Vern Gambetta, a well-known author and coach who has consulted with many sports, responded to a Twitter post by asking 'What is performance therapy?', and his follow up question was 'Why?'. Clearly these are important questions, which I will do my best to provide definitive answers to here.

PERFORMANCE THERAPY IN PRACTICE...

To define 'performance therapy' it is a useful to provide an illustrative example of an environment where performance therapy is a part of everyday practice. My visit to the Altis training centre in Phoenix in late 2015 provided such an example. Performance therapy is a cornerstone of the Altis approach; treatment tables and therapists are a permanent fixture on track side at every session, and the treatment rooms at the strength training facility are similarly fully staffed each afternoon.

But what are the defining characteristics that separate this practice from what occurs elsewhere? What is the essence of what makes it 'performance therapy'?

> "I truly believe that mechanical efficiency can be affected daily by therapy inputs. Treat athletes like F1 race cars."

> — Dan Pfaff

DIRECTED AND INTEGRATED...

My original attempt at answering Vern's question within the 140 character limit was '...essentially directed track-side therapy'. This brings us onto the two key defining elements of performance therapy. The first is that it is directed (ideally by coaches who possess a highly developed eye for movement and the ability to detect normal vs aberrant function). The second critical feature is the immediacy and ready availability of therapy, both prior to and during practice and/or competition.

> "Remove the restriction to more optimal movement – don't try to exercise your way out of 'dysfunction'"

> — Stuart McMillan

In the training environment what makes it 'performance therapy' is the capacity for appropriate treatment delivered in a timely manner to positively influence the athlete's ability to perform the training prescribed on any given day. Therapy delivered in this way can have a significant impact on the quality of training performed over the course of a training block.

Performance therapy therefore has the potential to directly and positively influence progression and training outcomes over time. This exemplifies that timely therapy intervention can have a direct effect on training input, the training outcomes that result, and ultimately the athlete's performance capacity and capability.

Where this expertise is available, therapy can similarly play a highly complementary and potentially decisive role during competition. In this context, directed, timely and appropriate treatment intervention can have a direct and highly positive effect on performance in competition. For instance, relieving restriction and associated inhibition can positively impact upon the athlete's ability to function and their readiness to perform. Again, this describes the potential for a direct link between the application of therapy and performance.

Returning to the 'directed' aspect of performance therapy, the monitoring process that prompts and informs treatment intervention is incumbent not only on the coach but also the athlete themselves.

DAILY CALIBRATION...

And here we turn once more to Altis to provide a practical example of how this daily monitoring can be achieved. The warm up protocol performed by each squad is carefully devised to not only prepare the athlete to train and rehearse specific movement patterns, but more than this the exercises that comprise the dynamic warm up are carefully chosen to screen for areas of restriction and associated movement compensations. The coaches themselves not only actively observe the warm up each day, but also have a critical eye on their athletes for any other tell-tale signs from their posture, gait patterns or general demeanour from the moment they arrive at training.

"Constant critical observation of movement is an active skill"

— Stuart McMillan

But clearly the most sensitive detection system for any areas of restriction or altered function on a day-to-day basis is the athlete themselves. There should necessarily be an onus on the athlete to take responsibility for this. This is also a long term process to educate the athlete and develop their body awareness so that they are more attuned to their own posture and movement. Effectively the objective over time is to increase the sensitivity and specificity of the athlete's own self detection system.

HANDS AND EYES...

Finally the success of the performance therapy approach is ultimately dependent upon the practitioner. Clearly a necessary first step is for the practitioner to be able (and willing) to move beyond the confines of the clinic or treatment room and station themselves in the training environment to observe and to treat athletes. Part of this exposure to the training environment is to gain critical insight into not only athletic movement but also the nuances of movement for the sport.

> "Embracing a model where therapists spend time observing athletes in sporting movements is critical"
>
> — Gerry Ramogida

The availability of the practitioner at daily training is critical to ensure timely intervention. As mentioned previously, this is a key point of difference with the performance therapy approach. Whilst I dislike buzz words, performance therapy is by its nature 'pro-active'. Specifically, the intention is to pre-empt issues so that treatment is provided at the earliest opportunity before a 'minor' complaint or 'niggle' (restriction or altered function) leads to an injury episode.

WHAT ELSE, WHERE ELSE...

Similarly, when assessing the athlete, the focus of the practitioner must shift from solely treating the complaint to establishing and addressing the root cause. Clearly the affected area must be treated, but the practitioner must also discern symptoms versus cause, and take appropriate measures to address both primary and secondary factors.

Essentially, the role of the performance therapist is detective and 'fixer' in a pre-emptive manner, rather than merely a fire fighter tackling each blaze in a reactive fashion.

> "Don't just focus on the symptomatic area. Don't just focus on likely cause. Always think 'what else, where else'."
>
> — Dan Pfaff

LOOKING FORWARDS...

In this chapter we have attempted to capture the essence of 'performance therapy', and detail some of the points of difference that define performance therapy in practice.

Looking forwards, the uncommon skills and higher-level understanding of the performance therapist are likely to be an important part of the solution in the 'frontier territories' of injury risk management and return to competition, and pushing the boundaries of athlete preparation at the cutting edge of elite sport.

Section Five – Developmental Athletes

Perils of the Talent Label

A thletic talent and sporting potential are hard to define and harder still to capture. Such ambiguity presents a major obstacle for 'talent identification' and 'talent development' programmes in sport. Marking out a youngster as 'talented' is not only fraught with uncertainty, doing so can also carry negative consequences for their development moving forward. In this chapter we will explore the topic of 'talent' and discuss the challenges inherent in the processes of talent identification and development. In light of these issues we will examine how we might best nurture and develop young athletes whilst avoiding the pitfalls that can result from labelling them as 'talented'.

In a recent conversation with a colleague who works in the realm of talent development the central theme of our discussion and the single issue that most preoccupied her was how she might avoid the term 'talent'. My colleague is not alone in this: coaches who work in development pathways in different sports often speak about paradoxical negative consequences for those selected to squads and identified as 'talented'.

GIFTS OF PARENTAGE...

An alternative description of talent is 'giftedness'. This term perhaps better captures the essence of what we are describing when we say a youngster is talented athletically. Often we are referring to gifts bestowed at birth; in coaching parlance they chose their parents well.

As we will explore later in the chapter, lauding a young athlete for such gifts of parentage is a problem. By definition they have done nothing to earn these gifts or the plaudits that accompany them.

Nevertheless in certain sports and athletic events we must recognise that there are inherited traits which are essentially prerequisites for attaining elite level. Selection and success in these sports require certain minima with respect to height, limb length, or size. A male discus thrower who is not tall and does not have a large wing-span will struggle to throw world class distances. If your parents are both short (less than six foot) you are unlikely to play center in the NBA.

These examples illustrate that in certain sports and athletic events there is essentially a 'natural selection' process. Despite these considerations, inherited traits alone are not sufficient for success at elite level. This is the case even in sports that favour 'outliers' from the extremes of the 'normal' population curve.

Those caveats aside, we must recognise that the genetic 'gifts' of anthropometry, physical size, and physiological capacities (cardiac function, muscle fibre-type distribution) are factors that can allow youngsters to rise to prominence in many sports.

Inherited traits lead to natural affinity for certain activities; examples include jumping, running fast or running far.

Inherited traits also extend to an athlete's responsiveness to different types of training, such as strength training or endurance training, and also the ceiling for training adaptations. In his book The Sports Gene, David Epstein describes this phenomenon as the 'Talent of Trainability'. Broadly, individuals can be stratified into 'responders', 'non-responders', and 'super-responders'.

Genotype can be important to varying degrees according to the sport. Even so, the extent to which these genetic gifts are expressed - what we term 'phenotype' - depends upon the athlete's environment and activities undertaken during critical phases in growth and development. The term 'epigenetics' describes such environmental or non-genetic factors with respect to gene expression. Epigenetics are clearly critical from a 'talent development' viewpoint.

Moreover, the majority of sports are more 'complex' in that they are reliant upon technical, tactical and decision-making elements. Clearly this makes these sports considerably less bound by gross physical and physiological capacities. In these sports, inherited traits are far less a prerequisite for success.

TRUE 'TALENT' IS HARD TO IDENTIFY...

Given the complexity that is inherent in most sports, evaluating the propensity to progress to elite level is far less straightforward than simply picking out the giants among the group. Identifying 'talent' in these sports defies simple measurement.

It is more difficult still to discriminate potential champion performers from an immature group of athletes. Even within an age-group this is a heterogenous population; particularly prior to late adolescence young athletes will possess differing and highly individual growth, maturation and development curves.

Often those identified as 'gifted' at age-group level are simply at a more advanced stage in their growth and maturation. The child might be an early-maturer. Or it might simply amount to a happy coincidence of birth date in relation to the eligibility window for age-group selection within the sport.

The phenomenon of the relative age effect can be observed across sports in different parts of the world. Essentially those who are born at a more advantageous time within the selection window so that they are relatively older and more developed than their peers are consistently favoured in recruitment to squads.

Talent ID systems in sport are notoriously flawed and protocols employed typically demonstrate very poor predictive value [52]. It is true that there is a self-fulfilling element whereby being selected to talent squads affords opportunities and exposure to coaching not available to peers. However, despite such advantages the conversion from age-grade squads to senior level is very poor. In fact, talent ID and selection at junior-level is remarkable in its failure to capture the true essence that allows athletes to succeed long term - or even in the short term in many cases.

HAZARDS OF LABELING...

"You do not reward 'potential'; you reward achievement"

– Greg Hull

There are unforeseen negative consequences that can arise from identifying a young athlete as 'talented'. Often when a young athlete is told they have natural talent, you are describing physical attributes or inherited traits. This amounts to rewarding what has not been earned. In many instances the 'athletic talent' they are being congratulated for simply represents an accident of genetics. This has been more colourfully described as 'winning the sperm lottery'.

Whatever the origin of their talent, young athletes who are lauded as talented from an early stage in their development are often fawned over and granted privileged status. As we will delve into in the next chapter, privilege is not conducive to developing elite behaviours. Selection to a talent squad can inadvertently send a message that the young athlete has made it, which in turn can lead to them becoming unfocussed and complacent.

Such complacency is not conducive to mobilising the mental resources necessary for skill development. Young athletes who are heralded as talented can become sloppy. As we will discuss later in the chapter, for practice to be effective the athlete must be attentive and intensely focussed. If an athlete is going through the motions or mindless in their practice this will serve to retard their development.

Being identified as 'talented' can also have negative implications in a different way. For some the mantle of 'talented athlete' can hang heavy. For many young performers, their self-concept is closely entwined to their status as a sporting 'talent'. Ultimately this can be oppressive.

Naturally in such cases there will be a tendency for the immature athlete to seek to guard their 'talented' status. As a result, young athletes may become averse to challenge or situations in which they do not feel proficient or deem that there is a risk of failing. In particular, talented youngsters may develop an aversion to failing publicly. This is a problem; error is integral to learning and acquiring new skills. In essence, to develop you must be prepared to fail.

ASCENDING THE SUMMIT REQUIRES HERCULEAN APPLICATION...

In The Talent Code, Daniel Coyle makes a compelling case that 'greatness isn't born, it's grown' [53]. As we have discussed, for certain sports it is irrefutable that genetic traits represent important determinants for participation at elite level. The points made by Coyle nevertheless remain valid; biological constraints aside, ultimately success in any sport is built upon particular behaviours and other qualities such as tenacity.

Whatever natural talent or gifts the athlete brings, ultimately there are no shortcuts. Development is built upon quality actions repeated over time. Quality action is in turn dependent on the level of attention, specific intent and effort invested. Efficacious practice might therefore be best described as repetition of desired behaviours.

The aforementioned behaviours concern what effort and will the athlete brings to their practice. Not only does this require considerable investment of time, they must also be systematic in the process and completely invested in the pursuit. As we will see, for practice to be effective the athlete must be fully engaged.

What we are describing has been termed deep practice in Daniel Coyle's book. This is analogous to the concept of 'deliberate practice' proposed by Anders Ericsson. The distinction between simple repetition and deliberate practice whereby the performer is engaged with specific purpose and intent is an important one. Ericsson has proposed deliberate practice as the factor that differentiates the path to expert performance [54].

There is a neurological or biological basis for these governing principles of deep or deliberate practice. Essentially, there are certain conditions which must be fulfilled in order to lay down white matter (myelin). Myelination is the process of adaptation that comes from training the neural circuitry for a movement so that it adapts by adding layer upon layer of myelin like insulating tape around a wire. This is the infrastructure of well-practiced skilled movement.

Sport represents a series of problem-solving tasks. To improve and develop the athlete must be directed in their efforts to resolve the problem and willing to attempt different solutions, make mistakes and learn from them. They must be mindful and aware of errors as they occur, and use this awareness to come up with new solutions and refine subsequent attempts to eliminate those errors.

Skilled movement that appears effortless is the product of countless hours of effortful and mindful endeavour. An athlete who wishes to achieve mastery must be willing to invest themselves fully in the struggle. They must be prepared to grapple with the complexity of the task and commit to the pursuit over the long term. There are clear parallels here with the recent chapter on the differentiating factors of elite practice and behaviours in sport. The time and effort invested will ultimately bring its rewards with the adaptation of the neural circuitry that supports well-honed and skilled movement.

DEVELOPMENTAL 'WINDOWS'...

There are phases of normal growth and development where youngsters are particularly receptive to learning. It is erroneous to view these developmental windows as a temporary 'one-off' opportunity. The window does not close if you miss the respective critical period; it is still possible to acquire skills later in life, albeit the learning process does tend to prove more difficult.

Still, it is absolutely true that within these receptive phases of development children are particularly responsive to acquiring sports skills and athletic abilities. Once again, this can be linked to biological mechanisms. For instance, during these fertile times for skill-learning children possess greater resources for laying down white matter (myelin), which as we have spoken about is the scaffolding that skill is built upon. It follows that it is critical for long-term development that young athletes are exposed to rich environments for learning and appropriate coaching during these developmental phases in order to take full advantage.

TALENT HOTBEDS...

Talent hotbeds describe such environments that consistently produce an inordinate number of athletes who ascend to the top level in their sport. The sites of talent hotbeds around the world are typically unremarkable places at first glance. Often they do not boast great facilities and are not generally blessed with significant financial support. Indeed in most instances the lavish facilities, resources and extensive support staff of a 'high performance' or institute of sport set up are conspicuously absent.

From such humble beginnings, talent hotbeds have nevertheless captured the alchemy of culture, environment and coaching that fosters intensive and consistent development. In short, they have somehow created the conditions which ultimately produce champion athletes year on year.

During my time in New Zealand I was fortunate to observe a talent hotbed first-hand. New Zealand is a small country in every sense, and the talent hotbed in question comes from track and field athletics, which is a minority sport in the country. Nevertheless, at one shared facility in the suburbs of the North Shore of Auckland a young coach named Jeremy McColl has largely single-handedly built a talent hotbed that is becoming a conveyor belt of world class junior pole vaulters ascending to the senior ranks. The breakthrough performance to date was the Olympic bronze medal won at the recent Rio Olympics by 19-year old Eliza McCartney, competing at her first major outdoor championships as a senior.

The pole vault school that Jeremy has built shares the humble beginnings of most talent hotbeds; without any foundations of history or established success in the sport he has had to overcome shortcomings in facilities and equipment by building it himself. Another hallmark that is common to talent hotbeds is of course exceptional coaching, and this is also very much in evidence.

When spending time with the growing squads of youngsters that Jeremy coaches what is perhaps most striking however is their frame of reference concerning performance. Essentially the young athletes' collective perception of what is 'normal' is warped in the best way. Extraordinary performances have become viewed as an everyday event. Against this background, accelerated development and the meteoric ascent of youngsters who only recently took up the sport is accepted as normal and everyday. This is perhaps why all the members of the squad are so strikingly well-adjusted – it is hard to develop an over-inflated opinion of yourself when everybody else around you is assiduously going about their business of doing extraordinary things.

IN CLOSING: TALENT IS ELUSIVE...

The elusive nature of talent in sport defies most attempts to measure it. Whatever the physical capabilities required by the sport, objective assessments alone fail to capture the less tangible traits that ultimately allow athletes to progress to elite level. To date we have yet to find a more sensitive or specific instrument to detect the potential to excel in the sport than an experienced coach with an eye for 'talent' in the context of that sport.

Clearly it is important that youngsters who demonstrate potential are provided opportunities to develop. From this viewpoint, we must aim to create and maintain a rich learning environment that supports the ongoing process of acquiring and honing skills and athletic abilities. An essential element is for young athletes who show potential to be exposed to high-calibre coaching.

Beyond offering opportunities and coaching input, it is also critical to impose and reinforce standards of behaviour in order to support continued development. So-called gifted athletes need to be in an environment in which they are held accountable. Being indulged does not foster growth. On account of their gifts, it is also natural that elite young performers should be held to higher standards. Moreover self-awareness and unflinching reflection are critical elements that must be fostered if athletes are to progress.

Ongoing development is incumbent upon constant challenge. It is not enough to merely attend practice and perform repetitions of the movement. For an athlete to improve they must invest their full mental resources. They must be switched on and be fully dialled into the process. And they must have clear and specific intent.

> "Only those who dare to fail greatly can ever achieve greatly"
>
> — Robert F. Kennedy

Continuous improvement is contingent upon the athlete retaining a willingness to explore the limits of their capabilities. Young people can be reticent when it comes to standing out from their peer group, particularly in a public forum. Therefore it is critical to create an environment in which immature athletes feel sufficiently secure to dare to be exceptional.

Rewarding early success with privileged status risks making the athlete conservative and unwilling to jeopardise this status. Young developing athletes must be directed to remain forwards-looking, and constantly encouraged to relish the challenge of improving further. Fundamentally, athletes must also learn to accept that mistakes are integral to the process of learning and improving.

From this viewpoint, a fertile environment for development fosters a readiness to essentially fail; fail better...(repeat); ultimately conquer. This is the essence of the process of achieving mastery and virtuosity whatever the athletic or sports skill.

The Burden of Advantage in Athlete Development

The paradoxical burden of advantages is something that those who work with young athletes (and young people in general) often grapple with. We might consider this a 'first world problem of privilege' for developing athletes; some might even argue it is symptomatic of the wider ills of modern society. Whether or not you subscribe to such views, few would disagree that a sense of entitlement is the enemy when developing young people, regardless of whether the aim is that they grow up to become good people or top athletes. In either scenario, many of the qualities we are seeking to instill are much the same.

As we will explore in this chapter, the luxury of advantages, unless carefully managed, can pose a serious problem when our aim is fostering the traits necessary to strive for mastery and achieve long-term success in sport. We will investigate what makes a conducive environment for developing young athletes who demonstrate 'talent', and what pitfalls to avoid. Finally, we will tackle the question of how we might negotiate the challenges we presently face on our quest, and recommend practical steps to ensure young athletes are equipped with the fuel for the journey and the tools to overcome obstacles on the path to becoming elite.

'I BLAME THE PARENTS'...

There is a reason why kids who are continually indulged are described as 'spoiled'. Yet it must be stated at the outset that it is a gross oversimplification to place the full responsibility for our wayward youth on indulgent parents.

Particularly as they reach the teenage years, youngsters increasingly look to their peers as the example to follow, and peer approval increasingly vies for supremacy with parental approval. When considering social influences, we must also recognise that a significant portion of a young person's day is spent interacting with their smartphone or mobile device; this represents a potent and almost constant source of influence.

It is often said that kids are essentially a product of their environment. Taking a broader perspective, it becomes apparent that there are however a host of influences that are present in the home, school, social, and even online environment. Each of these influences contribute to shaping young athletes' values and behaviours.

When seeking to positively influence behaviours and instill good values, we must be realistic about the fact that very few of these influences are fully under the control of the coach, practitioner, or indeed parent.

FOSTERING TRAITS...

"I prefer to work with athletes who are passionate and driven about their craft. I like curious athletes... I enjoy athletes who live in gratitude and who are selfless with their time and friendships. There are very few lone wolf athletes at the top. In my experience the training group and culture defines the ceiling of performance."

— Dan Pfaff

In a previous chapter we have spoken about the perils of the 'talent' label, and how practices and systems employed to develop identified athletes can paradoxically have negative influence on their subsequent development.

As we will explore further in this chapter, presenting athletes who show promise with rewards of status and exposing them to a privileged existence is at odds with what is required to nurture their talent and develop the traits required to progress. Such issues are epidemic in youth academy systems in professional sports particularly.

So what are the characteristics of environments that demonstrate sustained success in this area?

CONDUCIVE ENVIRONMENTS...

Observers have identified that 'talent hotbeds' for the most part seem to exist in quite spartan settings, which are shorn of the trappings of 'high performance'. A common theme with these environments is the notable absence of the comforts of 'luxury' items, such as high spec equipment and teams of dedicated support staff on tap.

These observations would seem to suggest that a host of amenities and ready access to resources are superfluous to the process of developing athletes to succeed at elite level. We could even go further and consider the intriguing possibility that the presence of such superfluous items might end up being counterproductive. Certainly, as we will explore later in the chapter, the fact that successful environments are not built upon a system of external rewards is a critical factor in their success in fostering development and nurturing the intrinsic motivation that fuels this process.

Humble beginnings in fact appear to be a hallmark of successful environments that demonstrate sustained success in nurturing talent. Distance running culture in particular flourishes in a setting that lacks advantages, including what we might consider basic amenities such as transport. For kids who are raised in areas where there is no option but to run to school, running naturally becomes a way of life.

"Among the Kalenjin and Arsi tribes that traditionally produce the best runners in Kenya and Ethiopia, respectively, it is common for schoolchildren to begin distance running at an early age, both as a sporting activity and as the primary method of transport to and from school"

— Wilber & Pitsiladis [55]

EXPERTISE INVOLVES EFFORT...

Observing the practice habits of expert performers proves instructive. When athletes are allowed to self-select the skills that they practice it has been observed that intermediate-level athletes choose to practice the skill that they are proficient at. Conversely, the expert performers in the group chose to practice the skill they were weak at [56].

Many authors consider that one of the hallmarks of deliberate practice is that it is not inherently enjoyable. In the study of expert and intermediate performers, the expert athletes (who chose to practice their weaker skill) reported lower ratings of enjoyment during the practice session [56]. Once again, this supported the notion that two factors that differentiate deliberate or 'deep' practice is that it is effortful and not inherently enjoyable.

Intuitively, it makes sense that there will be an element of drudgery and struggle to invest time on a skill or area of performance that does not come easy to the athlete. Equally, what I often observe with elite performers is that they possess an innate drive to become better. Striving for mastery motivates much of the day to day behaviours of these individuals, and this is how they derive satisfaction in their work.

'DESIRABLE DIFFICULTY'...

A central theme of Malcolm Gladwell's book David and Goliath [26] is the notion of 'desirable difficulty' in developing successful people. Hereby a lack of advantages, or the presence of apparent disadvantages, paradoxically confers an advantage in the long run.

The concept of desirable difficulty was first developed by psychology researchers Elizabeth and Robert Bjork. One aspect of this idea is that impediments can serve to facilitate both the learning process and the outcome. With a nod to deliberate practice, and 'deep practice' as championed in The Talent Code [53], encountering challenges or difficulties forces the learner to engage in the process more deeply, tap into their reserves, and persevere.

In this way, the experience of difficulty actually creates conditions which prove more conducive to deeper learning and comprehension. Once they have overcome such difficulties, the learner's struggles are then also rewarded by superior retention and transfer of learning.

Clearly these ideas have implications for how we approach learning. Equally, these principles also apply to how we develop young athletes who show promise.

As has been noted, if you look into the back story of champion athletes, or successful individuals in any field, you will often find they have overcome significant life challenges on the journey to the summit. This is another theme that is central in Malcolm Gladwell's 'David and Goliath'.

Admittedly the 'talent needs trauma' narrative has proven to be slightly overblown, in the sense that it is not strictly necessary for an athlete to experience life-altering events in order to ascend to elite level. Nevertheless, subsequent publications agree on the benefits of exposure to 'real-life' challenges in the development process.

"If you find a path with no obstacles it probably doesn't lead anywhere"

— Frank A. Clark

Life experiences are as important for developing athletes as they are for producing well-adjusted humans. Just as trials and tribulations foster personal growth, the coping strategies derived during these struggles are also invaluable, and make for more resilient and self-driven athletes. In essence, the presence of obstacles on the path, and the ensuing struggles to overcome them, can ultimately pave the way for the athlete's success.

When we recognise the importance of life experience, exposure to 'real-life' challenges, and the value inherent in the process of overcoming these obstacles, once again it is apparent that developing athletes who live a privileged existence protected from these challenges are missing out on critical opportunities for growth. This represents an increasing issue as they ascend to higher levels of competition, in which the ability to respond to adversity understandably becomes a prized asset.

ADVANTAGES MUST BE MANAGED...

As noted, socio-economic and cultural factors are generally accepted to contribute to the success of East African nations in distance running. More specifically, central to this success is a lack of advantages, such that running is the default mode of transport for many of these societies. This is in keeping with the 'desirable difficulty' hypothesis.

In contrast, for European or North American kids whom we can consider affluent by comparison, there is often the option of being chauffeured to school by parents, or at least catching a school bus. Oddly enough, we don't see many of these kids running to school.

Here we can see that advantages associated with a relatively privileged upbringing, including ready access to labour-saving options, are not conducive to steering kids onto the path required for pursuits such as distance running, which by their nature require habitual hard work to attain success.

We should also note that this phenomenon is not limited to the western world. It has been noted that the children of champion Kenyan distance runners fail to reach same heights in the sport. The wealth of the parents and advantages it affords them (including being driven to school) are the very things that makes success unlikely.

These examples illustrate how an upbringing of relative affluence and environments that provide ready access to amenities can be detrimental to developing athletes. Advantages must therefore be managed if they are not to become an obstacle to achieving success. If we continually provide kids with access to the easy option, naturally this is the path that most will take.

POISONING THE WELL OF INTRINSIC MOTIVATION...

It is important to recognise that there are natural sources of motivation that are intrinsic to the task, and therefore require no external influence. Moreover, in the absence of external influence, such intrinsic sources of motivation can be endless. However, these natural wells of intrinsic drive to perform an activity must be carefully managed and protected. Societal influences and external factors can degrade these precious natural resources.

In contrast, environments built upon external rewards and instant gratification promote extrinsic motivation. What makes this damaging is that it is to the detriment of intrinsic motivation. This is a problem that is particularly prevalent in youth academies in professional sport where kids are exposed to rewards from an early stage. Even if young players are solely motivated by the love of the game at the outset, these rewards quickly threaten to extinguish intrinsic drive, so that extrinsic motivation (i.e. contingent rewards) becomes the predominant driver for many.

Due to the nature of extrinsic motivation, youngsters in these environments quickly become accustomed to such external rewards, so that they no longer hold the same value. As a result, drive wanes until we 'up the ante' by providing bigger rewards, which will work for a time, until eventually the process repeats itself.

Regardless of the sport, the path to mastery is long. Gratification and rewards associated with the outcome are by definition long delayed. Indeed, it is typically years before the rewards of the outcome are realised. Circumstances therefore demand that motivation must be derived from the process itself. In essence, for the most part the journey must bring its own rewards.

Once again, a cosseted environment and a culture of entitlement fosters a demand for instant gratification. If those leading the process submit to the pressure to constantly reward with positive reinforcement whether earned or not, the effects are often negative and lasting. Clearly these conditions are not conducive to the long journey involved when striving for mastery.

Whilst well meaning, indulging kids in this way is inevitably damaging to motivation, and tends to diminish the enjoyment that is inherent to the task. Clearly this does not lend itself to the young athlete assuming ownership of their own development, and accepting responsibility and accountability for the process.

CREATING AN ALTERNATIVE ENVIRONMENT...

One antidote for the perils of modern society is to strive to make the training or practice environment an oasis from the rest of the world. For teenagers especially there is great pressure to fit in and conform to what is popular. The training environment should suspend these pressures. In turn we can establish an alternative set of standards and behaviours that youngsters might not experience elsewhere.

Within the training environment, the young athlete should feel unencumbered about engaging in something that they care about deeply. The environment should also provide the security and freedom to stand out, so that they can grant themselves the permission to be extraordinary and pursue their own path.

A keystone of this process is creating an environment that engenders intrinsic motivation. Kids more than anyone are hard-wired to enjoy the process of solving puzzles. Kids like to be challenged, and enjoy exploring different solutions. We must therefore tap into that well of intrinsic motivation.

In order to achieve this end we must take advantage of the inherent value of the training task itself. From this viewpoint it is important how exercises are presented. We need make explicit what purpose they serve in the overall process; if they understand the value of the task they are more likely to invest themselves in it. Another key tool to foster engagement is to present and deliver training as a series of problem-solving tasks, rather than exercises being viewed as solely a means to an end. We must emphasise the inherent value in the process, above and beyond the outcome.

THE ROLE OF THE COACH...

The role of the coach or practitioner in first creating and then maintaining an environment that fosters growth is critical. From the outset, the coach must take the lead on defining standards and expectations. Thereafter, all coaches and practitioners on staff must actively develop and reinforce the culture, via their day-to-day actions, behaviours, and interactions with the athletes.

Given this pivotal role, each member of the coaching staff must be very clear on the specifics of their role in the day-to-day process.

Firstly, it is not the role of the coach to keep the young athlete happy. The role of the coach is to provide a safe environment that provides appropriate challenge. Delivery should be driven by what gives the best opportunity for the athlete to improve; the coach is not there to entertain or to indulge the athlete.

"Leadership is getting someone to do what they don't want to do, to achieve what they want to achieve"

— Tom Landry

As noted, we must be ready to challenge the young athlete. This applies not only to the training tasks set, but also upholding the standards of behaviour that are expected of them. There may be resistance to this. The coaching staff must enlist the parents as a key ally in this process. Without their involvement and parental backing for this endeavour it is likely to prove futile.

THE POWER OF PURPOSE...

Young people (and adults) possess an intrinsic need to feel they have purpose, and a natural desire to engage in purposeful action. Kids who are privileged and have fallen into a sense of entitlement are dissatisfied. That indulgence and entitlement do not bring them satisfaction should give us hope.

The pursuit of mastery can provide this purpose. By definition, mastery is a journey not a destination. Attaining mastery is essentially a process without end; there is always scope to get better. In turn, striving for mastery can provide a constant source of purposeful action, and inspire insatiable curiosity for the activity itself.

In the right conditions, working towards mastery provides its own rewards. Naturally, youngsters must choose wisely; they need to care enough about the sport or activity to want to invest their efforts in the pursuit.

TAKING ADVANTAGE OF CHALLENGING EXPERIENCES...

As we have spoken about earlier in the chapter, life experiences and exposure to real-life challenges can be an invaluable part of the athletes' journey. Equally important is how the young athlete responds to these challenges, as noted by prominent authors on the topic, including Dave Collins [57]. Indeed, one of the criteria that wise coaches employ when evaluating a promising athlete is how they respond to adversity.

It is apparent that there is value to be derived from encountering and overcoming challenges, not least in developed coping strategies, and enabling the athlete to become more resilient and better equipped to deal with future challenges as a result. It follows that setbacks and difficulties should therefore be re-framed as 'opportunities for growth'. As far as possible young athletes should therefore be encouraged to embrace the process of enduring and overcoming these challenges.

Given the value of these experiences and the apparent benefits they offer, some authors raise the intriguing suggestion of whether we can manufacture such opportunities, or creatively impose 'desirable difficulties' during the athlete development journey. This was the topic of a thought-provoking recent publication by Dave Collins and colleagues entitled 'Putting the Bumps in the Rocky Road: Optimizing the Pathway to Excellence' [57].

Sadly, contriving such challenges has to date too often taken the form of 'boot camp'-style workouts. Such practices in the name of developing resilience or grit are becoming commonplace in sport at different levels, including youth sport. For the most part these efforts might best be described as misdirected, and in the worst cases (including recent scandals) those responsible are guilty of wilfully exposing their athletes to harm. Aside from violating duty of care, this is clearly not conducive to earning the athletes' trust.

I would submit that, even among the most privileged youth, the young athletes' experiences in their sport, the preparation process, and their life outside sport will naturally offer a ready source of life experiences and 'real-life' challenges. It is therefore incumbent upon us as coaches and practitioners to be attentive in recognising these 'opportunities for growth', and counsel the athlete to make best use of these experiences when they occur. Our role is to facilitate, as opposed to intervening on their behalf, or 'protecting them' from these valuable life experiences.

POSITIVE 'SOCIAL FACILITATION'...

As Malcolm Gladwell notes in his popular text 'Outliers' [58], to explain the full story of the success of wildly successful people you must take into account not only the unique circumstances involved, but also the roles that culture, community, and societal influences play in the process.

If we can create the right training environment, we can harness the powerful effects of positive peer influence and peer-learning. One such example is that communal influences can positively impact the young athletes' frame of reference. As noted in a previous chapter, talent hotbeds are a great example of this, whereby kids in an environment where extraordinary feats are a daily occurrence become accustomed to this, to the extent that extraordinary levels of performance are perceived as normal and expected.

OWNERSHIP IN THE ATHLETE DEVELOPMENT PROCESS...

Parental support is a critical aspect in relation to athlete development. The role of the parent is often pivotal in providing opportunities to participate and engage in practices and training. Parents are often quite literally the driver, in the sense that they provide transport to training, practice and competitions!

However, the parent, or indeed any other external player, cannot become the major driver in the young athlete's journey. The young athlete needs to own the process, and be afforded an increasing level of responsibility in steering their own course. Deferring to their parents to drive everything is clearly contrary to the intrinsic motivation necessary to achieve in the long term.

Ultimately what will prove most decisive is how important the pursuit is to the athlete themselves. This is the key question that must be answered sooner rather than later, as it will determine the choices they make, and the actions they take.

IT IS A CHOICE...

The element of choice is something we need made make young athletes acutely aware of. They need to be clear that the choice resides with them. Equally, they also need to be clear on the importance of their choices, and what hinges on the choices they make.

The first step is to be clear and explicit about the fact that it is not enough to simply turn up. Attending training or practice does not automatically mean they will improve or adapt. It is what the athlete invests upon arriving at training or practice that ultimately determines the outcome.

Choosing to attend training provides the opportunity. Taking this opportunity involves further choices. Deriving the benefits each day hinges on the athlete's choosing to 'switch on' once they arrive, and remain 'dialled in' during the session. Once again, these are choices. Nobody can make the choice but the athlete themselves.

The actions and behaviours of the coaching staff are once again critical here. For instance, rewarding kids with a high-five simply for turning up is somewhat missing the point. Whilst it is critical that they first show up in order to give themselves the opportunity, equally they have not yet done anything worth rewarding.

"Never complain about the results you didn't get from the work you didn't do..."

— Anon

With choice comes responsibility. Young athletes must be made aware and held responsible for their role in the process; and in turn made aware and held accountable for how this impacts the outcomes of training. If they fail to attend regularly they rob themselves of the opportunity to improve. If the young athlete fails to engage fully in the training process each day, they fail to make full use of the opportunity afforded to them.

Young athletes need to have clarity about why they are there; and they need to remain mindful of this. In a later chapter we will speak about the importance of mobilising athletes' mental resources during training. Having made the choice to come to training, the athlete must still decide what attention, intention and directed mental effort they are going to invest in their training on that day. On a practical level, we must prompt the young athlete to ask themselves these critical questions each time they arrive at the training venue to encourage them to make better choices.

A Practical Take on Long Term Athlete Development

Long-term athlete development has perhaps never been more topical, with an ever-growing number of programmes worldwide providing training for children and adolescent athletes. Mostly there is agreement on the need for structured 'athlete development' programmes for kids who engage in youth sports. We have consensus that appropriate physical and athletic development is beneficial for kids' health, performance and long-term outcomes. Still, confusion remains among parents, young athletes and practitioners, as authorities in the field continue to hotly debate the details. Here we will attempt to cut through these debates and provide much needed clarity and context to resolve some of the confusion. As we generally agree on the 'why', we will attempt to move things forward by finding shared ground and common principles to guide the 'what' and 'how' in relation to long-term athlete development.

THE GOVERNING PRINCIPLES OF ATHLETE DEVELOPMENT...

As was aptly put in an excellent presentation by a friend and colleague, the focus for any athlete development programme should be the athlete. Whilst this might be stating the obvious, too often this is lost sight of by those involved in development pathways in the sport, and the growing number of 'talent' programmes at school, club, and representative-level.

So perhaps this merits repeating: the best interests of the individual (i.e. the child or teenager concerned) must govern all processes and decision-making in athlete development programmes.

Likewise, by definition, long-term outcomes must take precedence over short-term results. Hence, long-term athlete development. Once again, this is a fundamental premise that few would disagree with. And yet, the odds are those who have experienced youth sports will have observed instances where this principle is violated.

There are many cases of myopia in youth sports, chasing the win on game day with little or no regard for long-term perspectives. Indeed there are numerous examples in different sports where policy and age-grade competition structures directly contradict governing principles of long-term athlete development.

THE GREAT DEBATES...

Taking such contradictions in practice aside, few among the key 'stake-holders' (coaches, practitioners, parents, athletes) would argue against the governing principles of athlete development we have described. All parties would tend to agree that the approach should be 'athlete-centric' and prioritise long-term outcomes. So, what exactly are we arguing about?

Essentially there are three major areas of debate and disagreement in relation to athlete development.

The first major debating point surrounds the model or system that we should employ for long-term athlete development (I refer the reader to the chapter dealing with the topic of training systems).

The second concerns how we should assess or evaluate maturation, often termed 'relative' or biological age.

Finally, in various sports there are diverging views on specialisation (focusing on one chosen sport) versus 'sampling' (continuing to engage in multiple sports). For example, arguments remain on what age athletes need to choose to specialise in order to acquire mastery in a particular sport, and ultimately attain elite level in senior-grade competition.

DEBATE #1 - BATTLE OF THE 'ATHLETE DEVELOPMENT' MODELS...

Until recently, the long-term athlete development (LTAD) 'model', originally pioneered by Istvan Balyi, was the predominant and most widely accepted approach. For a number of years, the popular version of the LTAD model attributed to Balyi had been enthusiastically adopted by many national sporting organisations worldwide.

In the recent period notable publications in the sports science literature have raised questions over the LTAD model as commonly employed. These authors have highlighted flaws in certain aspects of the LTAD framework [59]. The empirical evidence underpinning particular elements of the model has also come under challenge.

Some of the authors of these publications have since proposed alternative models, including the Youth Physical Development 'YPD' model [60]. The implication is that the 'new' model proposed should replace to the 'old' LTAD model.

Such publications 'debunking' the established LTAD approach have therefore heralded something of a shift in popular opinion. To some degree there is a trend of rejecting the LTAD model in favour of alternative approaches which have risen to prominence (including the aforementioned YPD model).

It is important that flaws in the details of the existing popular 'LTAD' frameworks and associated methodology are acknowledged. That said, it is also critical that we stop short of discrediting the wider premise of long-term athlete development.

Clearly an unwanted outcome is that LTAD as a concept falls out of favour and becomes a discredited term among authors and practitioners in field. Flaws in the interpretation and application of the LTAD model should detract from the fact the fundamental premise and central tenets of the approach are sound.

HOW DO WE RESOLVE THIS..?

There are a number of parallels here with the present debates on training periodisation. In recent times John Kiely in particular has exposed the tenuous rationale for many of the popular periodisation models [24]. It is argued that much of what is proposed by conventional periodisation schemes is arbitrary and not grounded in physiology. However, even the most scathing critics of these periodisation models nevertheless agree on the need for planned and systematic variation in training prescription. This is of course the essence of what periodisation exists to provide. We are therefore debating the merits of the methodology and conventions that have become associated with the principle, rather than the principle itself.

Returning to the debates on athlete development models, legitimate questions have been raised over how the LTAD framework has been applied. The growing field of research in paediatric exercise science continues to generate new findings and data. These emerging insights indicate certain assertions of the original LTAD model to be somewhat flawed.

For instance, some (quite logical) assumptions on what training is appropriate at different developmental stages based on biological maturation and physiology have been dispelled. One such example concerns the stated position of the original LTAD model regarding the use of interval training in pre-adolescence. Prior to puberty, young athletes' capacity for glycolytic metabolism is not well developed; it seemed to follow that 'anaerobic' training modes like interval training would therefore not be appropriate. Whilst this was sound in theory, in practice it turns out interval training is actually quite effective even prior to puberty; the nature of the adaptations that result are simply different [61].

The reality is that any model will prove to have shortcomings over time as research fills in the gaps in our knowledge. Equally, taking a wider view (and as we have identified in a previous chapter) any system too rigidly and dogmatically applied will inevitably lead to flawed practice and adverse outcomes.

Much like Matveyev's linear periodisation framework, it should also be considered that Balyi's original LTAD framework was likely intended as an illustrative example, rather than a blueprint that must be strictly and religiously followed.

The concept of long-term athlete development has value. Putting another way, we might argue that the main value of long-term athlete development lies in its use as a wider concept. Once again, understanding principles allows us to select methods accordingly, rather than confining ourselves to a set approach.

We must also consider the fact that, however well-meaning, by introducing new terms we muddy the waters. Sports science and medicine are plagued by issues of nomenclature. A myriad of different terms exist in the literature that essentially describe the same thing; proposing a 'new' term (youth physical development) to rival the existing recognised concept (LTAD) is another example of this. Such issues of labelling present an obstacle and a source of confusion for the audience we need to reach (parents, coaches, and the athletes themselves).

There is a lot of value in the 'new' methodology described in the recent literature. That said, taking a wider view, it is crucial to recognise that proposing competing models to replace the LTAD model is more likely to divide opinion rather than moving things forward.

"It is amazing what you can accomplish if you do not care who gets the credit"

— Harry S. Truman

Allowing arguments on details of application and specifics of methodology to spill over risks the wider concept of long term athlete development becoming discredited in the eyes of practitioners, coaches, parents and athletes. It might serve us better to focus on the principles we share agreement on. Shared purpose will allow the practice conducted under the banner of 'LTAD' to evolve.

DEBATE #2 - METHODS TO ASSESS MATURATION...

The central issues concerning the assessment of 'biological age' or relative maturation in youngsters revolve around ethics and practicality. What might be considered best practice or 'gold standard' from an academic viewpoint does not necessarily equate with what is realistic in a practical setting. This is not a new problem. For instance, standard methods in paediatric research to evaluate maturation based on markers of puberty and secondary indices of sexual development, such as Tanner stages, have long been plagued with these issues.

Similarly, the present 'gold standard' measure of maturity involves assessment of 'skeletal age' via X-ray. Clearly there are issues of practicality with this mode of assessment, given the cost and difficulty getting access to specialist equipment and staff. There are also ethical issues of routinely exposing children to X-ray radiation without any medical cause to do so.

To safeguard both the child and the practitioner, indirect assessments of biological age are therefore the norm. Typically these methods yield predictions and estimates based on simple measurements, such as height and weight.

Age at peak height velocity (PHV) is one of the more popular 'field' assessments, based on measurements of body mass and height, and using regression equations developed by Mirwald and colleagues [62] to derive individual estimates for males and females, respectively. The reference point used for the maturity estimate is 'peak height velocity' - i.e. the steepest portion of the growth curve corresponding to the greatest rate of growth in height. This 'PHV' reference point is more commonly termed the 'adolescent growth spurt'. The 'maturity offset' values derived therefore refers to the how many (decimal) years the individual is away from this reference point. For instance, +1.1 years indicates that the individual is 1.1 year past the age they are estimated to have hit their adolescent growth spurt (age at PHV).

The regression equations developed by Mirwald and colleagues [62] are based on the original growth curve data of a sample population of children and adolescents in Canada. More recent attempts to validate these regression equations in other populations in different parts of the world have reported discrepancies in predicted versus measured values for the respective populations. This is not entirely unexpected. Naturally, genetics will differ between populations, and environmental influences on growth and development inevitably exist in different parts of the world.

Another potential issue recently reported with this method is that the degree of prediction error may depend on the athlete's age and how close they are to their adolescent growth spurt at the time of assessment.

In response to the issues and sources of prediction error identified in the literature, some authors are steering away from Mirwald's age at PHV assessment in favour of other approaches.

One of the alternatives being championed involves prediction of adult height and related estimates based on standing height data recorded from both biological parents. It should however be noted that this method may also prove problematic, depending on different factors such as the particular family circumstances of the young athlete.

CAN WE FIND RESOLUTION HERE..?

An important starting point is to recognise that any indirect mode of evaluation represents a compromise. By definition any indirect method has limitations; this is accepted because it also provides a pragmatic means to gather data, avoiding ethical and practical issues.

The other governing principle in choosing an indirect measure of biological age is to consider how we will apply this information.

Let me give you an example. The approach I developed for the athlete development programme I was previously involved with in New Zealand was based upon three 'bio-banded' tiers. These bio-bands are quite broad. For instance, as depicted in the figure below, the middle tier is around 2-2.5 years in 'width'. The lower and upper tiers are broader still, encompassing quite a wide range in terms of chronological ages.

| **Pre PHV** | **>0.5 years prior** to estimated age @ PHV |

- Discovery, Exploration, Interaction
- Learning, Acquiring Capability

| **Mid PHV** | **<0.5 yrs pre to 1.5/2yrs post** estimated age @ PHV |

- Relearning, Recalibrating, Refining
- Developing Capability

| **Post PHV** | **>1.5/2 yrs post** estimated age @ PHV |

- Challenging Capability
- Developing Capacity

Figure 7: 3-Tier 'Bio-Band' Approach

With this approach, athletes' maturation assessment data is employed in two ways. The first is to guide which of the three tiers each new athlete is assigned to upon entry to the programme. The second application is as an objective means to track readiness to transition to the next stage, or 'bio-band', as the young athlete progresses over time.

Once again, the structure of the programme dictates what we need from the maturation assessment. Returning to the 3-tier 'bio-band' athlete development programme outlined above, given the broad groupings employed we essentially just need our maturation estimate to identify which 'ballpark' the athlete is in. For instance, if we were employing more narrow bio-banded grouping were more narrow (e.g. 1-year increments), there would be a need for 'higher resolution' - demanding a greater degree of accuracy and narrower confidence limits from the measure chosen.

As it stands, the mode of assessment I personally choose to employ involves the aforementioned Mirwald regression equations. Along with date of birth information (captured on entry to the programme), we periodically measure body mass, standing and seated height to derive the measures we need to input into the respective equations for males and females.

At this stage we should note that it is perfectly acceptable to use the alternative method that derives estimates from (biological) parental height data. Other programmes in different parts of the world choose to use this method. Once again, it comes down to preference and individual judgement. You simply need to weigh up practicality and logistical factors. And of course we should consider context, particularly with respect to how the data will actually be used.

There are other important points to note here. Whilst the athlete's maturation data is considered when assigning an athlete to a respective bio-banded group, or deciding whether to transition them to the next stage, equally it is not the only information considered.

Firstly, the assessment process is not a single snap shot: we continue to take serial measurements to track changes in height over time. Consider a young male who is estimated to be at a biological age marking him as ready to transition to the upper bio band. If his serial measurements - and my own observations - indicate that the athlete is still growing at an accelerated rate then we will not transition him, regardless what the maturity assessment indicates.

This example illustrates the second important point: it is incumbent upon the practitioner to interpret the maturation data derived for each athlete. Once again, it is critical to consider context, and be mindful of the limitations of the assessment mode and 'confidence limits' of the estimates derived.

Returning to the programme I previously ran in New Zealand, clearly we must bear in mind that the demographics of the population are somewhat different to the original Canadian sample the regression equations are derived from. A related consideration is ethnicity. Once again, a limitation of the regression equations is that it will likely cope less well with ethnic groups other than white-European. On that basis, I interpreted the values derived with a great deal of caution when assessing Maori or Pasifika athletes, those of Chinese or Korean descent, etc.

DEBATE #3 - SAMPLING VERSUS SPECIALISATION...

Our final point of contention differs somewhat to the debates described previously. On the topic of early specialisation most authorities in the academic fields of paediatric exercise science and long-term athlete development are largely in agreement. The risks of early specialisation with respect to overuse injury and restricted development are well documented. Conversely, the potential benefits of sampling a diverse range of sports during the developmental years are widely identified.

The discrepancy here relates to what is overwhelmingly recommended, versus what can practically be achieved or supported when faced with the realities of competitive youth sports in the present era.

Let us state from the outset that the arguments in favour of 'sampling' multiple sports in preference to concentrating on a single sport (i.e. early specialisation) are many and all very sound. Not least from the viewpoint of developing global athleticism (see the earlier chapter defining what constitutes 'athleticism'), the potential benefits of exposing a young developing athlete to a wide and diverse array of sports and 'movement environments' are considerable.

HOWEVER, as stated, there are also some realities to face here. There are numerous examples of youth sports which now afford the opportunity to practice and compete year-round. Given these opportunities exist, we must consider that many kids will choose to engage in these sports year-round, regardless of what may be recommended. For these kids the time left over to participate in other sports is likely to be severely restricted.

One illustrative example is ice hockey in North America. In the past, ice hockey was a seasonal sport. For instance, if you grew up in Canada you would play ice hockey (perhaps outdoors) in the winter, and then find another sport in the summer months. Now there are organised spring/summer leagues, in addition to the main winter season, providing the opportunity to play (and be scouted) in the period in between.

However we might rail against this, often these are simply the realities we face. The growing number and severity of injuries reported in youth sports underlines that we must be prepared to move beyond the standard guidelines in these cases. For instance, it was reported recently that ACL reconstruction surgeries among children have tripled over the past 15 years.

Given the stakes involved, we must meet young athletes and parents where they are. To this end, it is time to propose compromise solutions to cater for those young athletes (and parents) who fall into this category of year-round single sport participation. What is recommended as the 'ideal' for the majority, i.e. sampling a range of sports perhaps until late in adolescence, may also not be manageable in practice or even beneficial in some instances.

IS SAMPLING ALWAYS THE ANSWER..?

A strong case for 'sampling', or multi-sports participation, can be made from a physical development, motor learning, and even psychosocial development perspective. However, this does assume that there is spare capacity in the young athlete's schedule to accommodate adding other sports.

There are certain practicalities to consider when attempting to participate in multiple sports. For instance, practices and competition seasons for the respective sports may overlap. Inevitably there will be some trade-off involved; generally something has to give. Whatever might be recommended, often what is sacrificed is adherence to physical preparation sessions. In this case, participating in additional sports is unlikely to bring the desired benefits if it is at the cost of being able to fully participate in general physical development.

Finally, we must also be mindful of managing overall load - and the how it is distributed within the week. Once again, the potential benefits must be weighed up against the risk of overwhelming the athlete and predisposing them to overuse injuries that are common in this population.

We must therefore consider that there will be cases where the young athlete's existing scholastic, sporting, physical preparation and other commitments simply do not support adding another sport.

ALTERNATE ROUTES TO PROVIDE 'DIVERSIFICATION'...

The major benefits of sampling from motor development and sensory-perceptual perspectives stem from providing the athlete with a variety of movement challenges in different environments as they grow and develop. Ensuring continued exposure to a wide 'bandwidth' of movements and interactions during these key developmental years is critical to foster global development of athleticism, and ultimately acquire a wider array of skills and abilities.

The question therefore is whether we can provide this diversity of motor development and sensory-perceptual challenge in another way?

Outside of sports participation, an alternative vehicle for providing the necessary diversity is the other training or physical preparation that young athletes might undertake alongside their sporting activities.

This alternate route will necessitate shifting the emphasis of physical preparation programmes delivered with youth sports athletes. At the outset we must re-frame the overall objective. It must be clear and explicit that the priority outcome is global development of athleticism, rather than more narrow goals which are bound to the sport or to the weights room.

Having clarity on the ultimate objective and associated outcomes will then inform our approach when training young athletes, as outlined in a previous chapter. In particular, physical preparation sessions should encompass a range of activities and challenges; and these should also deviate from what the athlete is exposed to elsewhere, such as in their sport. Hereby we can provide the requisite diversity of input and challenge to stimulate global development of athleticism.

Clearly how this is communicated to the athlete, parent and coach is critical. Sport-specific youth training programmes clearly will not fulfill the need for diversification; equally from an engagement viewpoint it is crucial that we make a compelling case for this approach. Once again, we return to the need for long-term perspectives which take precedence over short-term outcomes and associated metrics. By happy coincidence, in the short- and medium-term this approach will however also help safeguard against injury and allow the young athlete to perform better in whatever youth sport they are engaged in.

BRINGING IT ALL TOGETHER...

Having delved into the great debates of long-term athlete development, hopefully we are now closer to a way forward. Whatever the issues with the original model proposed, LTAD is an important concept and we must consider the consequences before we discredit the term. As our understanding improves, the methodology should be allowed to evolve and the rationale employed revised and updated without abandoning the concept and governing principles of LTAD altogether.

Pragmatism should also guide our selection of maturation assessments. Whichever method is chosen the limitations should be considered and the data interpreted in context. Ultimately it is up to the practitioner to apply whatever data is available to the programme in question, and use their own judgement to make informed decisions.

Finally, whilst it is important we remain vigilant to the dangers of early specialisation, we must also do what is necessary to reach our audience. Continuing the theme of pragmatism, where the realities of the situation demand it, we must be ready to move beyond blanket recommendations to propose alternative solutions. Where the young athletes schedule makes participation in multiple sports problematic, we should consider our approach to ensure the necessary diversification is provided in the physical preparation they undertake.

Solving the Puzzle of Training Young Athletes

A famous and often cited quote in relation to training youth is that 'children are not mini adults'. Clearly the approach to physical preparation for children and adolescents should differ to what is employed with athletes competing at senior level. This is evident from biological, physiological and long term development perspectives. What is less clearly defined are the specifics of how our approach should differ, and how things will alter according to the respective phase of growth and maturation. In this chapter we will aim to shed some light on this topic.

A UNIQUE OPPORTUNITY...

The opportunities afforded within this critical period to shape the young athlete are remarkable, due to the favourable interaction of training with natural growth and development that serves to augment adaptations. Within these critical development windows the young athlete is also highly responsive from a motor learning and neuromuscular development perspective. I would argue that such scope to profoundly impact the athlete's physical and athletic development never arises again in their career.

Arguably the necessity for structured physical preparation and athletic development programmes has also never been greater.

REVERSING THE TREND...

The early development of fundamental motor skills occurs by children interacting with their environment through active play. Essentially a youngster's movement skill playbook is developed from the exploratory process of jumping on and off things, running around, negotiating obstacles, throwing objects and catching them.

Recent trends among youth worldwide have seen a decline in active play; and this is evident in declining levels in children's mastery of fundamental movement skills (locomotion, jumping/landing, throwing/catching). There is also an indication that an increasing number are failing to meet the required threshold levels of physical activity to support normal growth and development [63].

Given that basic athletic movement skill development can no longer be assumed it is easy to make the case that age-appropriate youth training should essentially be viewed as a prerequisite for kids to participate in youth sports safely and competently [64]. Moreover, regular exposure to physical preparation during the developmental years may also be key to ensure the young athlete attains their genetic potential.

Equally, the risks of getting it wrong are also greater when dealing with young athletes. The prevalence of various overuse injuries in youth sports [65] and associated dangers of early specialisation [66] are widely documented in the sports medicine literature.

Clearly coaches and practitioners involved with youth sports must remain vigilant. It is critical when programming and delivering physical and athletic preparation to be highly aware of the stresses that young athletes are subject to, particularly in critical phases in their growth and maturation.

TAILORING OUR APPROACH...

Long term athlete development perspectives also point to the need for the structure of sessions and objectives of physical and athletic preparation to shift as the young athlete develops. Using the example of track and field athletics, a renowned authority in the sport named Frank Dick describes a progression to guide session design and outcomes for each stage of the pathway to senior level competition [67].

Recognising the importance of first enthusing children in the sport and helping to ignite the long term passion required to keep them involved, the objective in the initial stages is 'Excite to Participate'.

Similarly the next stage, 'Participate to Practice' identifies that kids in essence just want to get involved and have a go at the different activities. This should therefore be the emphasis in the early stages, rather than a focus on formal instruction and heavily structured sessions.

As the athlete matures and progresses the next stage described is 'Practice to Prepare'. This is the first time the young athlete is exposed to structured training and practice. Equally, the emphasis is motor learning and developing capability, rather than volume or intensity.

At the appropriate time, the focus will then shift to 'Prepare to Perform'. As the label suggests, at this stage the athlete will be challenged to a greater extent in their physical preparation. In the case of strength training, this will involve appropriate progression of load and exercise prescription. Nevertheless, the focus should remain on sound movement; the objective therefore is that the athlete's fundamental movement capabilities are robust under load. In doing so, capacity will increase, along with various strength qualities.

DEMARCATION...

But how do we delineate between each respective stage? The major criticism of popular long term athlete development models is due to the rigid and narrow demarcations in relation to training suitability recommendations according to chronological age. There are two glaring issues with this.

Firstly, chronological age is not a good indicator as it fails to account for early versus late maturers; young athletes of the same chronological age can vary widely with respect to where they are on their individual growth curve.

Secondly, the data does not support the narrow chronological age 'windows' of trainability that are often presented in long term athlete development models. Whilst the mechanisms for training effects and adaptations that take place will vary according to age and stage of maturation, a particular form of training (for instance interval training) can still be successfully applied at these different phases.

Biological age estimates offer a more appropriate means to compare and group individuals. In recognition of this, in recent years there has been a shift to 'bio-banded' junior competitions in different sports (notably soccer) employing biological age groups rather than chronological age. Individual growth curves vary, but the reference point employed (peak height velocity) is able to account for this. Peak height velocity literally means the greatest rate of change in height in a calendar year. Biological age is therefore expressed in relation to this reference point on the growth curve – i.e. PHV plus or minus years.

A PRACTICAL SOLUTION...

In the previous chapter we introduced a 'bio-banded' training approach employing three broad tiers: Pre-PHV (all ages up to 0.5 years prior to estimated age at peak height velocity); PHV (minus 0.5 years to 1.5-2 years post estimated age at PHV); and Post PHV (minimum 1.5 years post estimated age at PHV).

As we spoke about, regression equations exist [62] that allow indirect estimation of age at PHV for males and females, respectively. These equations require only four items of information that can be easily gathered from the athlete: date of birth; standing height; seated height; and body mass. These values can be input to derive estimated age at peak height velocity. Serial measurements can be used to refine these estimates.

Whilst we can make a strong case for youth training programmes, it is nevertheless critical that the focus for such programmes remains global physical and athletic development, as opposed to specialised training for a particular sport. The perils of early sport specialisation have been highlighted from a number of perspectives [68]. A central premise is that participating in a single sport from an early age may in fact be detrimental to overall athletic development.

DIVERSIFICATION...

Taking a longer term perspective the benefits of sampling a number of sports during the developmental years are increasingly recognised. A good analogy for the developing athlete is 'buffet not binge' - i.e. exposure to a wide and diverse array of sports is likely to develop a broader and deeper athletic playbook in the long run.

In the same way, it is vital that young athletes receive a varied and balanced 'diet' of training items and are exposed to a variety of activities that challenge them in different ways.

An overarching objective should be to develop adaptable athletes, who are capable of applying their physical capabilities and athletic skills to a variety of challenges - including other sports. Importantly this will also provide the option of switching to a different playing position or another sport at a later stage.

FINDING A PATH...

So practically what does this mean for how we approach physical preparation and athletic development at each phase? In the second part of this chapter we will explore how the approach to different tenets of training shifts as the young athlete advances through each of the major stages in their development.

A useful framework with respect to athletic development is the concept of 'affordances for action' [69]. The central tenet here is that the athlete perceives their environment and any objects or other players in a way that is scaled to their own body and limbs. By extension, what available actions are 'afforded' by the environment is perceived in relation to their own perceived capacities and capabilities.

PRE PHV PHASE...

As mentioned previous the process of exploration and interaction with the environment is critical to the early development of motor skills. For young athletes in the 'Pre-PHV' phase of their development, sessions will often be designed to allow them to actively explore different movement solutions as they negotiate different movement challenges and obstacles. Such a discovery-based learning approach that often involves active play working within certain constraints is therefore the focus at this stage.

A key outcome during this phase is developing 'movement dexterity'. Gymnastics provides a great tool here. Regular exposure to a variety of floor-based gymnastics working in different planes and axes of movement helps the young athlete develop awareness of dynamic position of their body and limbs in relation to the ground and in three-dimensional space during different activities.

That said, there will be a motor learning emphasis when introducing strength training movements, and this will necessarily involve instruction on fundamental movements (squat, lunge, step up etc) to give the young athlete clarity on what 'shapes' they are aiming for. For the most part, strength training only involves light implements. Appropriate use of implements facilitates learning and acquiring the 'feel' of the movement; however the athletes own body mass remains the major resistance that they overcome during training during this stage.

MID PHV PHASE...

The critical mid-PHV phase marks the introduction of more structured physical preparation. There is a neuromuscular training emphasis, particularly during strength training. As such, proper form and movement quality is the critical outcome or key performance indicator during sessions, rather than intensity or volume. Coaching delivery must be highly responsive during this period as neuromuscular function can fluctuate markedly, even day-to-day, particularly during periods of accelerated growth. This necessitates a high coach-to-athlete ratio during sessions to provide the level of individual attention required.

Similarly, the objective during athletic development sessions (jump/plyometrics, speed sessions, gymnastics sessions) is essentially to allow the young athlete to relearn, refine, recalibrate movements as they grow and their limbs and torso dimensions change. Returning to the concept of affordances, the athlete's interactions with their training environment during this phase can be viewed as a continuous process of exploring their changing capabilities and broadening their understanding of the movement strategies and task solutions available to them.

POST PHV PHASE...

Once growth curves stabilise and the young athlete makes the transition to Post PHV, the focus switches to building capacity in order to continue to develop capability. Practically what this means is that sessions in this phase will subject the athlete to progressively greater challenge. For instance, progressive overload becomes a greater feature during strength training sessions, albeit the key performance indicator will be that technique and movement quality remains robust under load. Similarly, the intensity and neuromuscular challenge will be progressed during athletic development sessions. A progressively less constrained approach therefore allows the young athlete to explore and express their developing power and speed capabilities.

BULLET PROOFING...

Finally, the other major objective of youth training is to develop athletes who are resilient to injury. Our aim is to build athletes who are physically robust and possess the athleticism to safeguard against injury. In turn, the 'anatomical adaptation' (strengthening of skeletal structures, connective tissues) and greater strength reserve developed will also allow them to recover more quickly when injuries do occur.

It is here that sport specificity does need to be accounted for. That is, we need to be aware of the characteristic stresses and risks of particular injuries the young athlete is exposed to in their sport(s); and ensure that appropriate counter-measures are implemented in their physical preparation.

A WAY FORWARD...

So there it is, not only are children not mini adults, youth training programmes also need to adapt their approach to physical preparation and athletic development in a way that is appropriate to where the young athlete presently sits on their individual growth curve. In practical terms, there are straightforward indirect means to assess biological age and stage of maturation. This chapter has also presented some practical guidelines on how the approach to each tenet of training will change as the young athlete advances through each stage in their development.

Training youth sports athletes clearly poses some unique challenges; however the rewards can be extraordinary.

Part Three: The Role of the Athlete

Section One – Managing Body

Self-Therapy Tools for the Athlete's Kit Bag

I read with interest an article entitled 'Iliotibial Band Syndrome: Please do not use a foam roller!'. The author of this article is esteemed sports physician Andrew Franklyn-Miller. I moved away from using foam rolling some years ago, so it was interesting to see this. There is some data to support the efficacy of self-massage using a foam roller to improve range of motion and other functional measures. However, by its nature the foam roller is a blunt tool. Applying compression over such a large area, the foam roller is too imprecise to be useful for self-myofascial release via trigger point therapy. Moreover, excessive and non-selective use of foam rolling has the potential to cause more trauma to the tissues than good. This discussion also prompted this chapter and the one that follows - if not the foam roller, which of the growing array of self-therapy and recovery tools on the market is worth the investment and space in the athlete's kit bag? In the next chapter, we will explore in more detail how to best use those tools that make the cut, with some examples.

ITEM #1 – BACK BALLS

The first item for the kit bag is commercially available as a single piece of kit that comes under a variety of names and different suppliers, but for the purposes of this chapter we will term them 'back balls'. The use of this self-therapy device has become quite widespread in recent years, but was originally pioneered in Australia by sports physiotherapist Mark Alexander, and has won the endorsement of the Australian Physiotherapy Association. In the next chapter we will explore in detail the different applications, but briefly this device is used to mobilise adjacent vertebrae and release surrounding structures by lying supine atop it, so that pressure is applied using the athlete's own weight. The device is positioned at the junction between each vertebrae, moving in turn from S1/L5 to upper thoracic/lower cervical region (stopping at C7-T1).

Whilst this equipment can be bought as a prefabricated single-piece device, a do-it-yourself version can be made very simply and inexpensively - quite literally comprising two balls in a sock. When trying this out for the first time, you might want to use relatively softer and more compressible balls - tennis balls or similar. However, most athletes who are accustomed to deep tissue massage and performance therapy will soon graduate to something harder and less easily compressed. I favour lacrosse balls as they are very firm but have a thin rubber outer shell which makes it less uncomfortable against the skin.

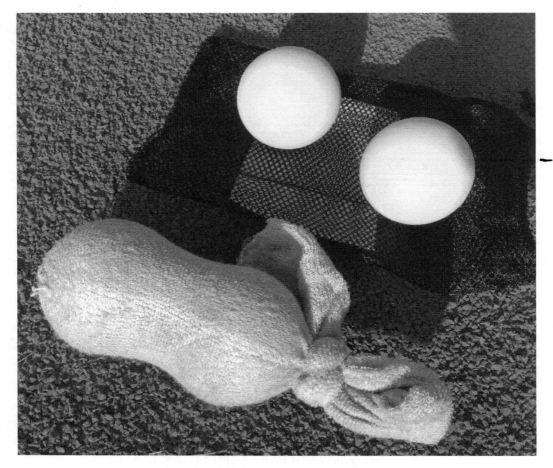

Figure 8: Self-Therapy Tools - 'DIY Back Balls'

Aside from being less costly - a legitimate factor in itself for many athletes - the DIY option has the advantage of being easily disassembled to provide the athlete with another self-therapy tool. The balls themselves can be employed to great effect for self-myofascial release or trigger point massage. Once more the lacrosse ball is superior for this application, being firm but with an outer coating that is 'nonslip' - almost as if it was designed for the purpose. Likewise due to its shape the ball provides a focal point that can be easily manoeuvred to apply pressure to the precise region of the myofascial trigger point. This is clearly not something that can be achieved with a foam roller. Using this simple tool, the athlete can also replicate modified versions of active release techniques.

ITEM #2 – YOGA STRAP

The second piece of kit that makes the cut is the humble yoga strap. This is another very inexpensive, light and very portable piece of equipment that can be employed for a variety of uses (as we will explore in more detail in the chapter that follows). One such application is as a tool for various mobility and assisted flexibility exercises for upper and lower limb.

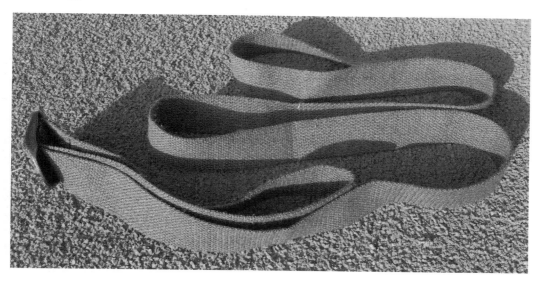

Figure 9: Self-Therapy Tools - Yoga Strap

The fact that the strap is made of inelastic material, and can be easily adjusted and fastened in a loop, also allows it to be employed to provide static resistance for isometric efforts (both submaximal and maximal). This application is particularly useful for the muscles of the hip. Similar 'activation' exercises for the gluteal muscles has been documented to serve an apparent potentiating effect when employed prior to dynamic activities such as jumping.

For instance, a study by Crow and colleagues [70] employed exercises recruiting the gluteal muscles in a group of elite team sports athletes alongside vertical jump testing and reported improved jump scores immediately following. Isometric exercises using the yoga strap such as a resisted clam shell might therefore be employed in a similar way to serve an 'activation' and potentiation function prior to training and competition.

ITEM #3 – HEAVY RESISTANCE BAND

The heavy resistance band is a slightly more specialised piece of kit, but it is equally widely available from a host of different training equipment suppliers. To be used most effectively the band needs to be anchored to something immovable, such as a post or some wall bars - generally something suitable can be found at the training or competition facility. That said, there are also partner-assisted variations that can be employed with the help of a coach, therapist or training partner.

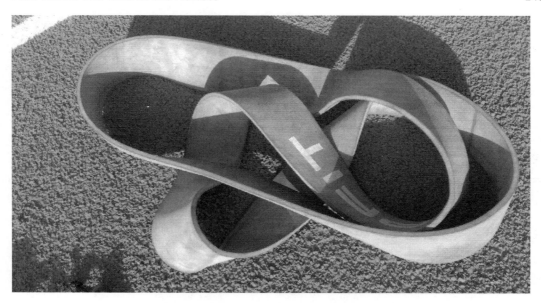

Figure 10: Self-Therapy Tools - Heavy Resistance Band

One of the major applications of the heavy resistance band from a self-therapy viewpoint is to provide traction to restore more normal joint function and mobility. For instance, conservative treatment modalities described in the sports medicine literature for hip impingement syndromes [71] include exercises that involve 'distraction' applied using a belt – or in this case the heavy band.

For athletes who require a high degree of hip mobility (hurdlers, jumpers, racquet sports players, ice hockey players), band distraction mobilisation techniques can be used in a pre-emptive fashion as a normal part of athletes' mobility work.

So there it is, a light-weight, inexpensive, and portable selection of self-therapy equipment that can be carried in the athlete's kit bag each day at training or when traveling to competition. In the next chapter we will describe in greater detail the different applications of these tools, with examples for athletes to try at home...

Self-Therapy Tools — What, When and How

More enlightened training environments (notably Altis in Phoenix) are throwing light on the benefits of ready access to performance therapy on a daily basis at the training facility. Whilst a growing audience is taking note, the reality for the majority of athletes is that they remain in less evolved systems and training environments that lack this provision. For the unfortunate majority self-therapy tools offer a substitute to hands-on manual therapy. In the previous chapter we made the selection of what self-therapy tools merit the precious space in an athlete's kit bag. In this chapter we will now discuss the what, when and how.

As we will explore, these tools have various applications in different instances. We will introduce some sample techniques and exercises to illustrate these applications and also to help guide athletes seeking to use these tools to best effect.

Due to the paucity of empirical evidence, these discussions are largely based on examples of best practice from leading practitioners and training environments, albeit we will touch upon what information is available from the sports medicine literature.

THE TOOL BOX...

Let us recap the items that made the selection from part one. Front and centre, the make-your-own back balls (constructed from lacrosse balls and a sock). Item two is a standard yoga strap made from inelastic material with an adjustable locking buckle. The final item was a heavy resistance band.

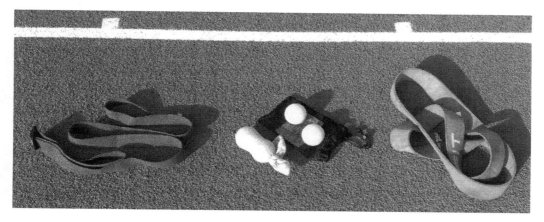

Figure 11: Self-Therapy Tool Kit

BACK BALLS...

The back balls are the first item out of the bag. A friend and former colleague (a sports physiotherapist named Chelsea Lane who at the time of writing is serving as Head of Physical Performance and Sports Medicine for Golden State Warriors in the NBA) has a strict rule that she will not allow any athlete under her care to lift until they have utilised the back balls in their warm up.

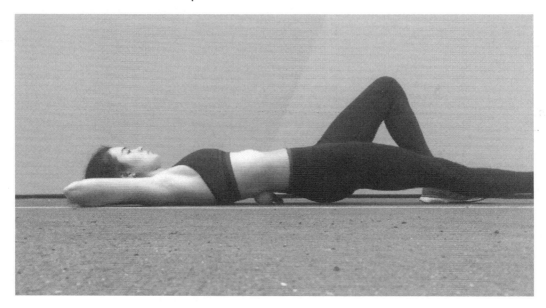

Figure 12: Back Balls in action

Accordingly, the athlete's routine upon arriving at the training facility or competition venue should be to spend some time on the back balls, working all segments from junction between lumbar spine and top of the pelvis to the top of the shoulder girdle (STOP there - i.e. avoid the neck). Adding (gentle) flexion/extension movements with either leg can also encourage the respective segments to mobilise. Similarly, by shifting to one side the back balls can also help to provide trigger point release for the muscles and connective structures adjacent to the spine.

The back balls are similarly a critical tool when the athlete is in transit, particularly on long haul flights. I would strongly encourage any athlete to pack the back balls in your hand luggage and take any and all opportunities to use them whilst waiting for flights. Similarly, the athlete should be diligent about using them once they have arrived at their destination to help work the kinks out before attempting to train or compete.

YOGA STRAP...

Item two, the yoga strap, can be employed for a variety of functions. For instance, as we spoke about in part 1, this offers a priming tool for the muscles of the hip girdle. Once adjusted, the athlete can perform isometric efforts at 90-, 45- and 10-degrees.

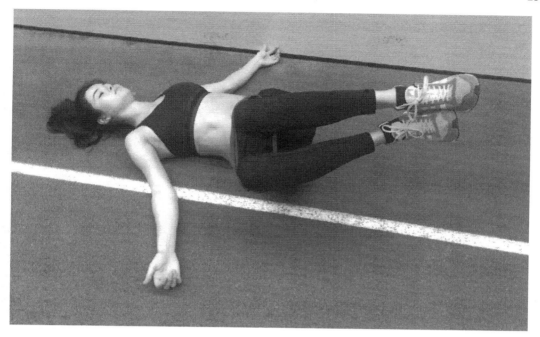

Figure 13: Using the Yoga Strap

With the same set up the athlete can also perform hip rolls to mobilise the thoracic spine, whilst maintaining tension against the strap and therefore activation of abductor and external rotator muscles of the hip. Once again, this is performed at both 90-degrees and 45-degrees.

Note that these are just a couple of examples of applications for this piece of kit. The yoga strap is similarly a great tool for mobility work for the shoulder girdle, particularly for athletes in racquet sports, contact sports, aquatic sports. Likewise, the strap can be employed to assist when performing flexibility exercises for both upper and lower limb.

HEAVY RESISTANCE BAND...

The final item in the self-therapy kit bag is the heavy resistance band. As well as a training device this is a great tool for mobilising the foot/ankle complex. This technique is particularly useful for track and field athletes, for whom foot/ankle mobility and impingement issues are relatively more common. Anecdotally, running-related conditions affecting the foot/ankle complex such as plantar fasciitis can also respond very favourably to this form of self-therapy, as part of the wider treatment regimen and reconditioning regime.

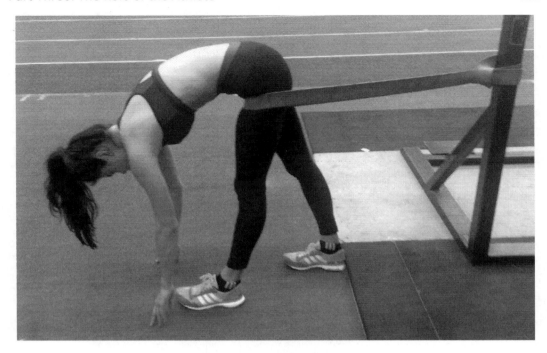

Figure 14: Heavy Band Hip Distraction

The heavy band is also a particularly useful therapeutic tool for the hip girdle. Athletes in a variety of different sports will be familiar with symptoms that fall under the umbrella diagnosis or syndrome termed femoral acetabular impingement (FAI).

> "'FAI' is an anatomical variant, a morphological state often related to imposed demand. It is hardly a diagnostic term.
>
> — Jas Randhawa

Given the prevalence of conditions diagnosed as 'FAI' in many sports (including among young athletes) conservative management that includes manual therapy is increasingly promoted, particularly in cases where there is no secondary joint damage that necessitates surgical intervention.

The major objective of the conservative management employed is to improve joint function. To that end, manual therapy often comprises joint mobilisation to provide more normal joint spacing and restore posterior glide of the head of the femur in the hip socket. To assist, traction may be applied in a lateral or posterior direction during hip joint mobilisations.

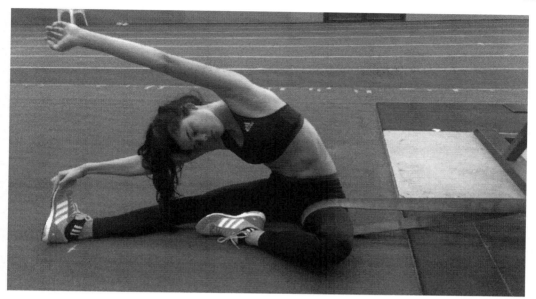

Figure 15: Heavy Band Lateral Hip Distraction

The heavy band can be utilised in a similar way to provide traction during self-therapy. Heavy band distraction is employed in appropriate postures and as an adjunct to flexibility exercises in a way that may offer relief for these symptoms and acute improvements in function. In much the same way as with standard manual therapy, this type of self-therapy can hereby serve a critical supporting role in enabling the athlete to perform the necessary training to improve the strength and dynamic stability afforded by the muscles of the hip.

Self-therapy when employed in this way can thus support and facilitate the intervention that provides more lasting improvements in function and symptoms.

IN SUMMARY...

So there we have it, some examples of daily applications of the self-therapy tools we selected for the athlete's kit bag. These tools and self-therapy techniques are particularly useful when applied alongside a daily mobility and pre-workout routine that serves as a self-screening or monitoring tool for the athlete. We will explore this practice and provide some examples in the next chapter.

Daily Mobility Series and 'Self Screen'

F or many years I have employed a mobility series prior to each day's training. Over the period I have refined the selection, and as we will see the mobility exercises employed borrows heavily from yoga. This practice is designed to serve two distinct purposes. Clearly one key objective is to prepare the athlete for the session to come. The second function is to allow the coach, practitioner and the athlete themselves to discern how their body is moving on each day. In turn this can serve to guide any self-therapy or performance therapy intervention needed to address the area of restriction or altered function detected during the course of the athlete's daily mobility routine.

A 'LIVE' MOVEMENT SCREEN...

This practice is far from unique - many top coaches and practitioners, particularly in track and field athletics, customarily employ mobility exercises as part of the warm up prior to each daily session. Moreover, variations of the exercises employed have been a part of practice in pursuits such as yoga for centuries.

> "Your warm up should be your living movement screen"
>
> — Gerry Ramogida

A notable example is Altis, a track and field facility and education centre in Phoenix, where the warm up routine is designed to serve as a daily screening process. The protocols employed by each of the coaches at Altis features an element of mobility - the selection of exercises may differ somewhat but mobility remains a key theme.

BUCKING THE TREND...

In other sports, notably team sports, the use of mobility exercises prior to training and competition has perhaps fallen out of favour due to the fear of blunting speed and power expression with the use of static stretching.

There are a couple of important points to note here. First, mobility exercise are somewhat distinct from static stretches in that the athlete actively moves themselves into the postures, and indeed in many of the mobility exercises the athlete is actively weight-bearing. In this sense, mobility exercises can more accurately be categorised as dynamic flexibility.

Moreover, the mobility routine is followed by the dynamic part of the warm up that comprises drills and other activities (e.g. running, jumping) of increasingly intensity. This second point is important to note. When we examine the studies reporting a blunting effect is observed following stretching, this effect is not only transient, but more pertinently appears to be eradicated when the stretch protocol is followed by dynamic activity [72].

SELECTING MOVEMENTS...

With respect to the selection of mobility exercises, as the pictures illustrate a key theme is spine mobility, or more specifically the articulation between each part of the spine, and associated structures - in particular pelvic girdle and shoulder girdle.

It is also important to note that these movements and postures involve not only musculoskeletal structures, but also connective tissue and myofascial structures. For instance, a number of the exercises involve different portions of the thoracolumbar fascia that serves as a corset and natural back belt, in addition to providing points of attachment for numerous muscles of the shoulder girdle, trunk and hip complex. For these reasons some have taken to 're-branding' such mobility exercises as 'fascia stretches'.

MOVEMENT QUALITY FOCUS...

What is optimal with respect to range of motion will differ according to the sport or athletic event, and will also depend upon the functional anatomy of the individual. Therefore it is the quality of the joint articulations, and the coordinated function and motion of the respective structures that is the focus.

As such, rather than emphasising range of motion, the key indicators are rather the quality of the motion and how evenly the range of motion is 'shared' between each segment of the kinetic chain. That said, we can expect there to be some level of chronic adaptation in response to this daily practice, so that improvements in mobility (i.e. active range of motion) will be observed over time.

> "What is your ideal monitoring system? Coaches that pay attention"
>
> — Dan Pfaff

DAILY 'DIAGNOSTIC' AND SELF-CALIBRATION...

By extension it follows that the most sensitive 'detection system' for any areas of restriction or altered function is the athlete themselves. Practitioners speak about athletes who are 'body aware'. This can be further defined using such terms as somatic awareness, proprioception and kinaesthetic sense.

Whilst it is critical that the coach and practitioner remains diligent about observing the mobility routine each day (and the dynamic warm up that follows), the athlete is also an active part of the process of detecting and notifying what they are feeling and any perceived restriction or altered function.

With mindful practice on a daily basis the athlete can become more highly attuned so that they are better able to discern daily changes. Over time we therefore observe that athletes become better able to self-screen with a greater degree of sensitivity and specificity. The mobility routine thus serves as a daily calibration.

TUNING IN...

Mindfulness is a key element in this process. Given that the athlete is the critical player in the process by extension it is hugely important that they are fully invested in the process and 'tuned in' when they complete this routine each day. Clearly there will be very little sensitivity in the detection system and very sloppy calibration if the athlete is not paying full attention and taking appropriate care with how they are performing each exercise.

Conversely, when the athlete is fully engaged in the process and in their daily practice, the mobility routine can be a highly effective tool to help the athlete to 'tune in' and enhance their mental and physical readiness for the training session to follow.

FINAL THOUGHTS: GAME DAY 'RITUAL'...

Over time the mobility series that the athlete settles on essentially becomes a daily ritual that serves an integral part of the athlete's physical and mental preparation. At competition time this ritual of familiar practice becomes highly valuable to the athlete, providing something to focus on and welcome diversion from anxious feelings and distracting thoughts, thereby serving a tool to help combat pre-competition anxiety.

You Must Have Good Tyres – Why and How to Train the Foot

Aside from serving as the point of weight-bearing for all activities performed in standing, the foot represents the terminal link in the kinetic chain where forces generated by the athlete are transmitted to the ground beneath them. The action of the foot is integral to all modes of gait, from walking to sprinting. During sprinting, for example, the athlete's technical proficiency in how they apply force during each foot contact is recognised as paramount. Despite the integral role of the foot in locomotion and a host of athletic activities common to the majority of sports, training to develop this critical link is often overlooked in the physical preparation undertaken by athletes. This chapter examines the role of the different muscle groups involved in the dynamic function of the foot. We will explore different training modalities to develop the respective muscle groups, and also discuss the applications of this form of training, from both sports injury and performance perspectives.

COACHING WISDOM…

"You Must Have Good Tyres"

— Jacques Piasenta

Jacques Piasenta may not be name known to many outside of France, and the sport of track and field athletics, but he boasts a long and distinguished career as a highly successful coach and trainer to multiple medallists (sprints and hurdles) at Olympic Games, World Champs, and European Champs.

Piasenta's quote captures the importance of the foot - the analogy of the tyres of a race car, or perhaps a motorcycle, is well chosen. The dynamic function of the foot is critical in relation to balance, traction and propulsion. Likewise, just as a racing team would not concentrate their efforts on the engine and neglect the tyres, it follows that it makes little sense to train each of the proximal links in the lower limb kinetic chain and then ignore the terminal segment that connects with the ground.

FOOT FUNCTION…

The functional anatomy of the foot is adapted to its various functions in standing and during gait, from balance and weight-bearing to shock absorption and force transmission during locomotion. The specialised architecture of the foot comprises arches of bones (longitudinal, or front-to-back, and transverse, or side-to-side), reinforced by both passive ligamentous structures and the dynamic support provided by myofascial structures (notably the plantar fascia) and a variety of muscles.

These ligament springs and elastic myofascial components allows the foot to function in a 'sprung' manner - deforming under load before springing back to its original shape. This compression and recoil action is important as it serves to first store and then return elastic energy during locomotion and other activities, such as jumping. The contribution of this elastic energy return to the overall mechanical energy expended during running for example is significant.

One important aspect of the dynamic action and functional anatomy of the foot during gait relates to pronation during gait, particularly when running. Specialised running shoes designed for 'pronation control' are a common site in running shoe shops. Many athletes will be familiar with the notion of being classified as an 'over-pronator'.

We should recognise that pronation is a naturally occurring action during gait that serves an important function. Whilst this is acknowledged in the literature, hyper-pronation is nevertheless commonly identified as a factor in numerous various overuse injuries of the lower extremity [73]. Clearly we need to distinguish between pronation as a functional action, versus instability and dysfunction resulting in loss of structural integrity at the foot during gait and weight-bearing tasks.

An alternative view that might resolve the confusion proposes that the issues we see are actually a case of 'abnormal control of pronation' and 'reduced dynamic control' of foot posture, as opposed to 'excessive pronation' [74]. This perspective allows us to move beyond demonising pronation, or obsessing about the degree of pronation range the athlete exhibits, and rather focus on their ability to regulate foot posture in weight-bearing and dynamically control the timing and degree of pronation that occurs during ground contact, for instance when running.

Two things to consider (and evaluate) are the functional anatomy of the foot in weight-bearing, and the degree of dynamic control we observe during gait. These are different, and should be assessed independently. In particular, we cannot infer dynamic control based upon a standing assessment. This points to the need for assessment performed barefoot in standing (both bilateral and unilateral stance), alongside a dynamic assessment (also barefoot). Whilst it will depend on the sport, most often this will comprise a running based assessment.

THE CAST OF SUPPORTING MUSCLES...

The muscles of the foot include both the intrinsic muscles on the plantar surface (sole) of the foot, which originate and insert at different bony structures of the foot, and extrinsic muscles that cross multiple lower joints with the belly of the muscle above the ankle.

Different portions of the intrinsic muscles provide dynamic support to the bony and ligamentous structures of the foot. The action of these intrinsic muscles can alter the functional architecture of the foot, such as height or length of the foot arches. For instance, the role of the intrinsic pedal musculature in supporting the medial longitudinal arch of the foot, and in turn the dynamic function of the foot and lower leg, has been established [75].

The intrinsic muscles also provide stability to the foot and assist with static and dynamic balance. For instance, the recruitment of plantar intrinsic muscles increases under conditions that demand additional stabilisation – for example when standing on one leg [76]. Finally, these muscles play a crucial role in the transmission of forces during gait and weight-bearing activities. Given their role in the effective distribution of force and shock absorption during weight-bearing tasks, developing these muscles has the potential to reduce stresses placed upon bone and ligament structures.

The extrinsic muscles of the foot originate above the ankle and so cross multiple joints. As such these muscles essentially operate as long pulleys and their action produces movement at the foot and ankle. The extrinsic muscles are considered the prime movers of the foot, and the long toe flexors in particular are important in generating propulsion during locomotion. Equally the extensors of the toes – particularly the big toe – serve a critical role during gait, first preparing the foot for ground contact and then in the recovery action after 'toe-off'.

DYSFUNCTION AND INJURY...

Impaired or altered function of the intrinsic plantar muscles particularly is linked to abnormal foot functional anatomy and mechanics, including rearfoot alignment in weight-bearing [77]. Clearly if the stacking of the anatomical structures at the foot is altered this will impact the stresses placed upon these structures [78]. These stresses will also be transmitted up the lower limb kinetic chain, and so will have implications for other joints further up.

The integral role of the muscles of the foot in supporting the structural integrity of the foot is readily apparent [78]. A demonstration of this is that when activation of key muscles is reduced under experimental conditions via nerve block there are measurable changes in the stacking of bony structures resulting in altered rearfoot alignment [75]. Similarly, when these muscles become fatigued changes in the functional anatomy of the foot during weight-bearing (specifically 'drop' or displacement of the navicular bone of the rear foot) can be observed [73].

Dysfunction of the foot muscles is observed in different overuse injuries, in particular those suffered by runners. For instance, atrophy (wasting) of the intrinsic plantar muscles has been found in runners suffering with chronic plantar fasciitis [79].

THE CASE FOR TRAINING THE FOOT...

As we have seen the respective members of the cast of supporting muscles are not only integral to normal function, they are also important from an injury perspective. These observations point to a clear need for remedial training to develop motor control and capacity for the various muscles that support the foot as part of rehabilitation for injured athletes [80]. By extension, it follows that dedicated training to develop foot muscle function will play an important for athletes who are suffering with overuse injury, and those predisposed to these injuries based on assessment.

What is less recognised is the value of training the foot for healthy athletes. The wisdom of exceptional coaches like Jacques Piasenta aside, in general the case for training the foot for performance is rarely made. This seems a bizarre oversight given the critical role of the foot in essentially any athletic activity performed weight-bearing in standing. For so many actions in sport the foot is the interface between the athlete and the environment. This interface is not only where the athlete imparts forces to the ground, but equally where ground reaction forces are returned and transmitted in order to produce movement.

Neuromuscular control and motor skill aspects of the interaction between the foot and the ground during running in particular have been identified as a critical factor that differentiates elite performers from sub-elite. For instance if we take a 40m sprint, the orientation and magnitude of the ground reaction impulse of force applied during each step determines propulsion and therefore velocity [81]. Likewise, 'technical ability of force application' is identified as a critical factor for maximal velocity sprinting [82].

TRAINABILITY...

But are these muscle groups responsive to training? Well, importantly, the answer to this is a firm 'yes'.

A range of studies report significant improvements in response to a variety of training interventions for the plantar intrinsic muscles, the toe flexor muscles, and toe extensors. The muscles of the foot are shown to be highly responsive to training, and strength scores for the respective muscle groups increase with short-term training interventions. The various positive outcomes also include changes in the functional anatomy of the foot in weight-bearing (changes in arch height and length) and improved dynamic balance scores [83].

Returning to the case for training the foot for performance, more striking is that a range of improvements in athletic performance measures have been reported following different foot training modalities. Improvements in horizontal jump distance have been reported following a short-term toe flexor training intervention [84]. This is a notable finding as it suggests that training the toe flexors can help steer impulse of force applied to the ground in a horizontal direction, making it highly relevant to any athletic activity requiring horizontal propulsion, including sprint running.

APPROACHES TO TRAINING THE FOOT...

So, we have established that developing the muscles of the foot is important, and that these muscles are responsive to training. The question that remains is how practically should we approach training for the respective muscle groups of the foot?

One approach might be to simply train barefoot or wearing 'minimalist' footwear. Indeed there is some preliminary evidence that undertaking athletic activity in minimalist footwear might elicit some training adaptation in the foot muscles. One approach might be to perform a portion of the strength training workout barefoot - particularly for exercises that involve single-limb support, in view of the finding that plantar muscle activity is higher during such exercises due to the greater postural stability demands involved [76].

One caveat with this approach is that, as has been reported recently with barefoot running interventions, responses to barefoot training are likely to be somewhat mixed [85]. The effectiveness of simply training barefoot or in minimalist footwear is likely to vary according to the individual. In part this will depend on individual differences in morphology. However, what is also critical is the athlete's understanding of what they are attempting to achieve – i.e. what constitutes 'good foot posture' and 'sound' mechanics.

A major factor in relation to the efficacy of barefoot training is therefore the level of instruction or coaching input provided. This is a likely explanation for the differences between 'responders' and 'non-responders' when barefoot running programmes are implemented without instruction [85]. The important role of instruction and the neuromuscular skill component of training the foot are crucial themes that we will return to later in the chapter.

The concept of the foot-core was introduced by McKeon and colleagues [78], drawing parallels with the 'core' that encompasses the structures and systems of support of the lumbo-pelvic-hip complex. As I have written about previously, whilst it is firmly established and widely recognised, I find the term 'core' entirely vague and unhelpful in relation to lumbopelvic stability [86]. That aside, the literature on the 'foot-core' merits some attention.

A major strength of the 'foot-core' paradigm is its acknowledgement and emphasis on the dynamic and coordinated function of the myriad of connective tissue structures and collection of muscles which contribute to supporting the architecture and action of the foot. The authors propose the 'foot core system' system as comprising the interaction of active, passive, and neural-subsystems [78]. Equally important is that this paradigm emphasises that the particular contributions from the respective elements is dynamic and dependent upon the conditions and constraints of the task.

From a practical viewpoint, one of the critical aspects identified by proponents of the 'foot-core' approach is the need for specific retraining to develop motor control and capacity of the intrinsic muscles of the foot [78]. Another element these authors emphasise is the need for integration. For instance, in a rehabilitation context they advocate a progression from isolation exercises to 'integration exercises', which combine the action of both intrinsic and extrinsic elements of the active subsystem, and emphasise motor control and sensorimotor input (i.e. 'neural subsystem') [80].

GROUPING TOES AND EXERCISES...

With respect to targeted training interventions, we can employ a functional distinction so that the four toes outside the big toe are treated as a functional unit, and devise appropriate exercises. We can then deal with the movers of the big toe as a separate entity for training purposes.

Arguably this makes more sense than separating the intrinsic versus extrinsic muscles. Whilst some investigations have attempted to isolate the intrinsic muscles without extrinsic muscle activity, the merit and utility of this practice in a real-world setting is perhaps questionable. We can and should employ different measures to favour recruitment of target muscles (including specific plantar intrinsic muscles). However we do not need to limit ourselves by specifying that other (extrinsic) muscles cannot have any involvement. This is a more pragmatic approach than what we often see in a clinical setting whereby the objective is to isolate muscles.

The 4-toe grouping was employed in a recent study that combined flexor strength scores of the outer four toes (without big toe) [87]. Just as foot training in general is often overlooked, the outer four toes in particular are frequently ignored during training. This is somewhat baffling given their integral role in supporting the dynamic function of the foot, especially during gait.

During running gait for example, it is the lateral part of the forefoot, or 5th metatarsal, which should ideally contact the ground first, before a medial shift onto the 1st metatarsal at weight acceptance. This initial contact and subsequent transition or weight shift is key to the transfer of energy between the metatarsal phalangeal (MTP) joints and the arch during the stance phase. The plantar muscles of the outer four toes help to control this initial contact and transition. Moreover, these muscles contribute to regulating the arch compression or deformation that occurs during ground contact.

The practical importance of the contribution of the intrinsic muscles to dynamic foot posture is reinforced by the aberrant findings reported among those with running overuse injuries. The mechanics of initial contact and transition observed during ground contact are different to what is seen in healthy runners [88]. This is demonstrated in the finding that the degree of arch deformation is greater both in standing and during running gait among those suffering with chronic medial tibial stress syndrome [89].

One aspect we do need to examine is the instructions employed to preferentially select the intrinsic musculature during the foot strengthening exercises most commonly employed in a clinical setting. For instance, the recommended instruction during the 'short foot' exercise is to draw the heads of the metatarsals (long bones of the foot which join the toes) towards the heels whilst keeping the toes relaxed. A variation of this is instruction is to raise the arch of the foot, whilst keep the toes relaxed. Aside from being a bit mind-bending for most athletes, practically this is also very difficult, which can negate the effectiveness of the exercise and thereby harms compliance.

An alternative method of instruction that has been proposed [74] is to emphasise the action at the proximal joints, as opposed to curling the toes. This approach distinguishes the action at the proximal (metatarsal-phalangeal) joint, which is largely produced by the intrinsic muscles, versus movement at the more distal toe joints produced by the action of extrinsic muscles.

NOVEL APPROACHES...

As noted earlier in the chapter, the most common exercises for the intrinsic plantar muscles in the sports medicine literature are variations of the 'short foot' exercise, performed with the foot planted. These exercises are essentially isometric - i.e. involve static contractions with relatively little movement. Moreover these exercises are performed with body weight resistance only. Both of these aspects limits both the degree of challenge and potential for progression, and these factors are likely to harm compliance over time.

A suggested modification involves the addition of a heavy band to apply resistance in an inward or medial direction (the image to the left in figure 16). This variation still involves quasi isometric contraction, but there is additional work to oppose the resistance applied in order to maintain the shape of the foot arch. This favours the recruitment of the more oblique intrinsic plantar muscles.

As we have spoken about, a different approach to instruction is also recommended. The athlete should be instructed to emphasise the action at the proximal joint of the toes, which should allow the toes to remain relatively extended (rather than actively curling the toes).

The athlete is also instructed to actively extend first the big toe, and then the outer four toes (raise them clear of the floor), before spreading the toes to reset between each successive repetition. Here we are essentially integrating a selection of the lesser exercises for the plantar intrinsic muscles that have featured, albeit infrequently, in the sports medicine literature and in the field [90]. Specifically, the athlete essentially performs the first-toe extension exercise, second-to-fifth toe extension exercise, and toes-spread out exercise between each repetition. Each of these exercises has demonstrated effectiveness in activating the range of plantar intrinsic muscles that support the foot [90].

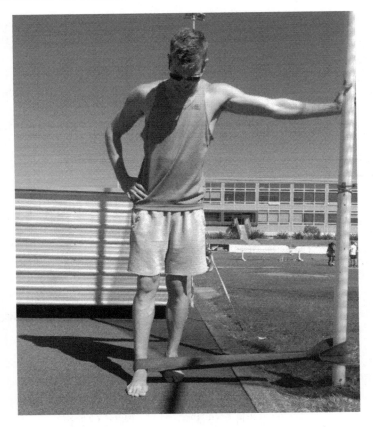

Figure 16 - Heavy Band Exercise for Plantar Intrinsic Muscles

Moving onto the big toe, we are not only concerned with the flexors and extensors, but also the muscles that produce lateral action at the big toe. It should be noted here that the proposed training modes are not isolation exercises; the other four toes are actively involved.

Training the short and long flexors of the big toe would seem to be a more straightforward proposition. In the field and in the literature this generally takes the form of exercises such as 'toe raises' and/or 'toe lowers', typically performed with body weight resistance.

A previous investigation established that the toe flexors produce the highest torques with the ankle in the range of 0-10-degrees of dorsiflexion (i.e. neutral and slightly flexed upwards) and the metatarsal-phalangeal joints (proximal toe joints) flexed within a range of 25-45-degrees [91]. These findings indicate that if our objective is to load the toe flexors then we should avoid any significant degree of ankle plantarflexion, as this requires the toe flexors to work at shortened lengths and therefore a mechanical disadvantage, reflected in greatly decreased torque generation [91]. All of which makes a strong case against relying on the standard toe raise, given that during this exercise the athlete moves out of the optimal ankle range from the outset, before working through full plantarflexion range. This is perhaps why the exercise is sometimes referred to as a 'calf raise'.

There is strong preliminary evidence that the toe flexors are highly responsive to strength training modalities that allow them to work within an optimal range to develop maximal torques [84]. The training intervention that has been reported employed a custom rig and involved isometric efforts.

Here we propose some variations with external resistance, to allow for progression and aid compliance over time. These variations also incorporate dynamic actions, combined with isometric efforts. The external resistance employs either resistance band, elastic tubing, or cable resistance anchored under the big toe to augment the degree of loading placed upon the toe flexors (figure 17).

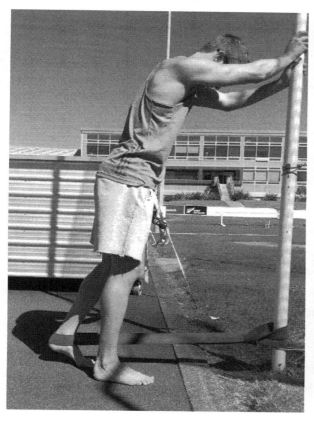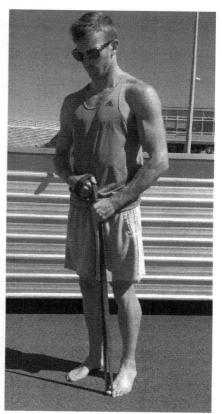

Figure 17: Resistance Band Big Toe Flexor Exercise

One of the featured exercises employs a heavy band. The athlete performs isometric efforts, first in the initial position and then in the terminal position, with concentric and eccentric efforts in the transition movements in between (pictured on the left in figure 17). In contrast to the standard toe raise exercise described previously, during which the ankle travels through a range of plantarflexion motion, in this exercise the ankle joint remains in a narrow range (from neutral to slight dorsiflexion) throughout. The toe flexors are therefore able to work in the ranges that provide the greatest mechanical advantage. In addition, these ranges correspond more closely to the joint angles that occur during the stance phase when running.

Once the athlete has mastered the basic techniques, progression for all of the exercises described can be achieved by shifting to a unilateral base of support; that is performing the movement supporting themselves on the resisted leg with the free leg unloaded. As we have spoken about previously, this alone will increase the activity of the plantar muscles supporting the foot [76].

As highlighted, we also need to consider the lateral movers of the big toe. For instance, abductor hallucis is a critical supporting muscle for the medial longitudinal arch of the foot. In addition to producing lateral (outward) movement, this muscle also contributes significantly to flexion of the big toe. Once again, we can increase the demand by using exercises that involve external resistance as the athlete attempts to move the big toe inwards (adduction) and outwards (abduction). Initially this might simply involve providing static resistance to work (isometrically) against. Over time, progressions might include more dynamic external resistance in the form of bands, elastic tubing or cable resistance.

Finally, the extensor muscles of the big toe can similarly be trained using equivalent exercises involving resistance bands or elastic tubing to provide resistance.

Essentially there are two main variations of toe extensor exercises. The first are isolation exercises that simply involve extending the big toe (i.e. raise the big toe upwards) under resistance whilst the foot (and other toes) remains planted. The band is held under the foot and looped around the top surface of the big toe. The second approach involves compound movements where the emphasis is maintaining the big toe in a flexed position as the lower limb moves through a range of movement. This is essentially the equivalent exercise to what is depicted in figure 16; however once more the resistance band is looped around the upper surface of the big toe, i.e. resisting extension rather than flexion.

MODIFIED DRILLS AND PLYOMETRICS...

Aside from resistance exercises, a variety of drills and low-amplitude plyometrics can also be employed to train the foot.

These drills are performed barefoot, or perhaps with minimalist footwear. Broadly, there are two main categories of foot conditioning activities.

The first category emphasise a bounce action, with minimal knee involvement, so that the emphasis is on the work occurring at the hip, ankle and foot. These drills are performed in multiple directions, with variations moving both forwards and backwards, as well as zigzag patterns and diagonal bounding.

One such example involves single-leg 'pogo' bounds in a lateral direction. The aim is for a rolling contact moving from near to far edge of the foot (in relation to the lateral direction of the motion). This rolling or 'wave' action recruits each of the toes in turn to generate propulsion in a lateral direction.

Progression can be achieved by extending the distance for repetitions and/or incorporating an incline slope. Resistance can also be added, for example holding a medicine ball. Other variations include performing these drills with resistance (medicine ball or barbell plate) held overhead.

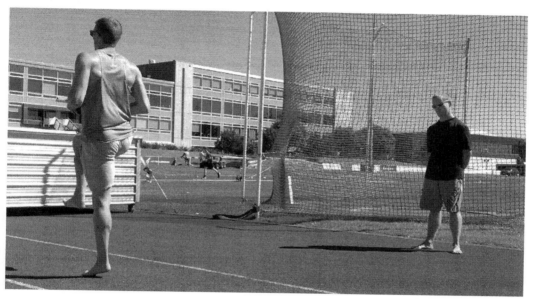

Figure 18: Low-amplitude Plyometric Foot Drills with Medicine Ball

The second category of drills are essentially modified sprint drills, which simulate more of a running gait pattern, with appropriate focus on foot contact during weight acceptance and propulsion. Once again, these drills are performed without shoes. The intention of the athlete is a large part of the neuromuscular training effect derived, so it is vital that these drills are instructed properly and executed correctly.

TAKE CARE OF THE TYRES...

So, there you have it – the 'why' and 'how' of training the various muscles of the foot, with a selection of examples and suggestions for effective training modes. As we have outlined, for athletes who run and jump it is critical to take account of foot strength and control in your training. After all, developing a big engine is ultimately futile if the tyres fail.

Section Two – Managing Mind

Mobilising Mental Resources

Ask any athlete or coach and they will readily acknowledge the mental side of training. The mind is an integral part of training the body. How an athlete perceives the training prescribed influences their experience of it. In turn this perception impacts how the athlete responds to the training performed. Despite their apparent importance, mental aspects of the training process are typically not accounted for in any structured or meaningful way. In this chapter we will elucidate what these critical elements or 'mental resources' are in relation to athletes' training. We will then explore how each of these aspects can be accounted for and harnessed to best effect in the way athletes' training plans are presented and delivered.

In a seminal publication, Ives and Shelley (2003) [92] introduced the notion of 'psychophysics' in relation to strength and power training. Specifically, the authors identified three key themes or psychological aspects pertaining to the training process:

1. Attention
2. Intention
3. Directed Mental Effort

Each of these aspects can have a profound influence during the training process, and in turn affect the outcome of training. We will return to this discussion and explore each of these aspects in detail later on in the chapter.

FIRST THINGS FIRST, ENLIST THE ATHLETE...

Firstly, and as we have spoken about in previous chapters, we need to conceptualise training as a process in which the athlete is an active player. This is an important distinction. Too often the athlete by default assumes a passive role in the process.

Redefining training as a process where the athlete plays an active role is therefore our starting point. In order to engage the athlete they must feel they are integral to the endeavour. Once the athlete feels like it is their programme, as opposed to the coach's plan, they are far more likely be fully invested and committed to the physical preparation prescribed.

By definition, each athlete is also the richest source of feedback and information available to the coach. Even under the same external load, each athlete's experience of a training session (i.e., 'internal load') is highly individual. Therefore, as coaches and practitioners we must also seek to enlist the athlete as an integral part of the ongoing monitoring and review process.

Clearly for all this to work the athlete must be prepared to take a level of ownership of their training. Equally they must engage in learning and invest the time to gain an understanding of the training process. With those caveats, the ultimate objective is that over time the athlete will become sufficiently involved and informed that they attain the right to directly input into the plan and the process of programming training.

TRAINING AS PROBLEM-SOLVING...

From a motor learning viewpoint any training task represents a problem-solving exercise for the athlete. Once again, as we have spoken about in previous chapters, this re-frames the role of the coach or practitioner as being one of a guide during the process. Essentially, the coach is there to define the task and associated constraints, and then assist the athlete in working through the challenge and figuring out solutions that satisfy the conditions imposed.

DEFINE THE TASK AND RELATED PARAMETERS...

The first objective of the practitioner is to provide clarity on what the task is. The most straightforward way of doing this is to first demonstrate the particular exercise. To complement this, the coach must then define the task in a simple and straightforward way that the athlete is able to understand and process.

Depending on the type of training, the bandwidth for what constitutes 'acceptable' execution of the task may be quite narrow; for instance, this is typically the case in the weights room. Conversely, for more complex athletic training there will be a variety of solutions that satisfy the constraints of the task, and greater scope for the athlete to explore the options available to them given their unique capacities and capabilities.

MAKE SURE THE ATHLETE IS CLEAR ON THE 'WHY'...

Once the athlete has a clear understanding of what the task is, and what constraints or conditions must be satisfied to execute the task successfully, the coach must promptly turn their attention from the 'what' to the 'why'. This point is often missed; however it is absolutely critical that the athlete is clear on the purpose.

Too often as coaches or practitioners we assume that the purpose is obvious; in essence, that it goes without saying. It can be highly instructive in these instances to ask the athlete what they think the purpose of the exercise is, or how it relates to their sport. My experience is that many times the athlete is not clear on the purpose or rationale, and this is the case particularly with younger athletes. On that basis, it cannot be assumed that the athlete understands the 'why'. Ultimately, there is very little that we should automatically consider goes without saying.

Clearly, it must be explicit what the function of the particular training is, and why it is important in the context of the athlete's sport and their specific needs or goals. Only once the athlete has a clear understanding of the purpose and how it relates can they be expected to fully invest their mental resources in performing the training prescribed.

Defining the 'what' and 'why' therefore both involve relating the task to what the athlete knows, and providing them with context of where it all fits with respect to goals and outcomes. Each of these elements are critical for capturing athletes' attention, which is the first of the three critical mental resources identified.

UNDERSTANDING PURPOSE CAPTURES ATTENTION...

Many authors in different areas speak of the importance of being 'mindful', or 'purposeful' in one's practice. By definition, the athlete must first have clarity on the purpose in order to be 'purposeful'. Likewise, it must be clear to the athlete why the training is important and how it will serve their needs and goals in order to capture their interest and attention sufficiently for them to be 'mindful'.

In addition to simply paying attention, the coach or practitioner can also steer where the athlete's attention is focussed. A number of studies [93] have examined the effects of directing a performer's locus of attention and what effect this can have on performance, learning, and retention. We will explore this topic in detail in the chapter that follows.

INTENTION DURING REPETITIONS AND SETS...

The second area where the coach or practitioner can provide direction on how the athlete executes their training is intention. The athlete's intent when they perform an activity is very powerful. Neuromuscular firing patterns are part predetermined in anticipation of the repetition [94]. Therefore intention can alter both the degree of muscle activation and motor patterns during the movement; and in turn what adaptations occur as a result [95].

Guiding the athlete with respect to intent, or setting them a specific objective when they perform each repetition can be powerful in directing their behaviour or output during the task. One example might be 'I want you to violently explode off the line and project yourself as far down the track as you can with each step' [96].

As you might imagine, providing cues of this nature to steer the athlete's intention when they perform a repetition of the exercise is likely to result in very different task execution or output.

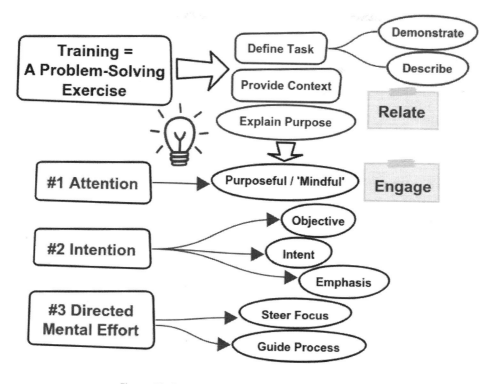

Figure 19: Attention, Intention, Directed Mental Effort

SHINE A TORCH TO STEER THE ATHLETE'S FOCUS...

Much like intention, it is important that the athlete not only summons the requisite level of effort during training but that this is also directed appropriately. Which brings us neatly onto the third and final mental aspect to account for and harness during training: directed mental effort.

Directed mental effort pertains to the degree of mental engagement in the task, and where they invest their mental resources.

As we spoke about previously in relation to attention, the coach can help direct the focus of the athlete's efforts to best effect during the training task. This mental effort might be directed towards a particular outcome, or to emphasise a particular aspect of how they perform the task.

IN CLOSING...

The three themes we have covered (Attention, Intention, Directed Mental Effort) will be important considerations regardless of the type of training involved. These aspects are applicable to all settings, from the weights room to a rehabilitation context.

As we have spoken about, attention, intention and directed mental effort should be considered when programming training. The themes should also be applied when presenting the session plan or introducing a particular exercise to the athlete. Finally, and perhaps most critically, these aspects should be accounted for in the way in which training is delivered and the coach's interactions with the athlete on a day to day basis.

There are a number of strong arguments to support that coaches in different sports and practitioners across disciplines would benefit from being aware and mindful of these aspects in their practice. Enlist the athlete, engage them in the process, and seek to apply the principles of attention, intention and directed mental effort to best mobilise athletes' mental resources and optimise training.

Locus of Focus – Where to Steer Attention

Locus refers to a place or position where something is located: locus of attention concerns the location of an athlete's focus when executing a movement. Typically, locus of attention is stratified into internally versus externally located focus. The current dominant message to coaches and practitioners is to cue in a way that avoids an internal focus of attention - essentially 'internal focus BAD; external focus GOOD'. Yet when we look beyond the dominant narrative and take a closer look at the research on the topic, the question of where and how to direct an athlete's locus of attention when learning and performing becomes rather more complex. There is growing evidence to indicate that what is optimal may vary according to the population concerned, the task, context and even individual preference or predisposition. In this chapter we will delve deeper and attempt to unravel the topic of locus of focus.

DEFINING EXTERNAL VERSUS INTERNAL FOCUS...

As always there is some distortion between research findings, the message that is portrayed, and what is ultimately received by practitioners on the ground.

On the most fundamental level, coaches' and practitioners' understanding of what constitutes 'internal' versus 'external' focus often differs to the definition in the literature.

As a first step, it would be useful to get some clarity on what exactly we are referring to when we say 'internal' focus versus 'external' focus. Understandably, most readers interpret internal focus as a focus on the athlete's own body, whereas an external focus could naturally assumed to be external to the body. Indeed a number of the studies in the literature have employed this distinction.

However, the most influential research group in the area of locus of attention employ a different definition. According to their definition, external focus is directed towards the movement outcome, whereas internal focus is directed to the process of the action itself.

Given different researchers on the topic are seemingly unable to agree on definitions, it is entirely unsurprising that there is confusion among practitioners and coaches working in the field.

For the purposes of this chapter, given we are speaking about locus - i.e. location or point in space of attentional focus - we will consider internal focus to be directed towards a specified area of the body during the movement, whereas external focus will be considered a particular location in the environment. That said, where research has used the alternative definition we will make this clear as we discuss the relevant findings.

Confused yet? Then let us proceed...

THE DOMINANT NARRATIVE...

By far the dominant narrative in the research literature and in the message presented to coaches and practitioners is essentially: 'internal focus BAD; external focus GOOD'. More specifically, the message is that coaches should avoid instruction or cues that direct the athlete's focus to an internal (bodily) location or aspect of the movement itself. Rather, instruction or cueing should direct the athlete's focus to a feature in the environment or the outcome of the movement.

There are two main reasons given why the external locus of attention approach is superior when learning and performing.

Firstly, when acquiring a skill if the athlete's focus is directed 'internally' to a body part or aspect of the movement skill this will result in 'explicit learning' focussing on the mechanics of the movement, whereas it is argued that the aim should be unconscious or implicit learning, fostering 'automaticity' of skilled performance. A side note, which is less often referred to, is that directing attention towards particular aspects of the skill might also constrain exploring different movement strategies when learning.

The second argument against internally directed focus relates to performing in a competitive environment. Here it is argued that internal focus is likely to encourage the athlete to consciously control what should be a relatively automated skilled movement. This tendency to revert to conscious control under pressure is termed 'reinvestment'. The argument is that internal focus, or 'self-focussed attention', leads to conscious control of movement mechanics; and this disrupts normal coordination, leading to inefficient motor control and compromising performance outcomes.

In summary, the argument is that internal focus should be avoided at all parts in the process. Adopting external focus when training is contended to provide more robust learning. External focus when performing will also combat the tendency to switch to conscious control under pressure and the associated negative consequences (often labelled 'choking').

A CLOSER LOOK...

A number of studies in the literature report similar findings in support of the consensus that external focus of attention is superior for learning and performance. So what is the problem? Should we not just take the locus of attention debate as resolved and heed the message that we must strive to avoid cues that encourage internal focus on body parts or movement mechanics?

Before we go ahead and dismiss internal focus entirely, let us conduct an exercise in critical thinking. Taking a closer look at the research on the topic, we find there are a number of factors to be considered...

DISCRIMINATING EFFECTS OF INSTRUCTION PROVIDED...

As is often the case, rather than taking the study conclusions or abstract at face value, it is instructive to take a closer look at the methodology employed.

In the interests of critical thinking we might consider the possibility that prominent researchers perhaps bring certain a priori judgements - for instance a theory they would like to see supported - which may influence the design and delivery of the research studies undertaken.

Specifically, if we look at the specific instructions given under the respective internal focus of attention versus external focus conditions this can be revealing. Indeed, examining these details may even lead us to possible alternative explanations for the findings reported.

There are a number of cases in the research literature where the instruction provided in the internal focus of attention condition are quite convoluted. In some instances they may also steer the learner or performer towards body parts or aspects of the action that are not entirely relevant or particularly helpful to successful execution of that task.

Consider this example from an investigation that employed volunteer novice subjects (aged 15-68 years):

> "As you are preparing to shoot the basketball try to think about your arm and wrist angles. Notice that when I bend my elbow I am forming a right-angle or 'L'? Think about this as you are shooting the ball. Also, think about your feet position and if you bend your knees think about this, too. Think about your body movements and angles.

— Weiss et al (2008) [97]

It is hard to discriminate in this example whether any difference in performance outcomes was due to participants' locus of attention, or simply a result of over-coaching and having been bombarded with too many cues, particularly given their level of experience.

Conversely, instructions provided under external focus of attention conditions in these studies are typically both more simple and more likely to direct the performers gaze to task-relevant information in the environment. For instance, in the same study: "focus on the basket itself or some other aspect of the immediate environment such as the front rim or backboard".

In any case, this does raise the question whether changes in performance outcomes reported in these studies are in fact due to internal focus of attention, or simply reflect the disruption and distraction caused by unfamiliar coaching cues or inappropriate instruction.

THE STORY WITH NOVICE VERSUS EXPERIENCED PERFORMERS...

As commonly occurs in sports science research, the majority of studies in this area have investigated novice performers rather than athletes. When investigations employ participants who are familiar with and skilled at the task being assessed the findings do not always follow the hypothesised universal superiority of external focus of attention.

There is growing evidence that the outcome may be different when high-skill performers execute the particular motor skill task under internal versus external focus conditions. When investigations employ experienced performers they seem better able to perform successfully using either internal or external focus of attention. They also appear more adept at switching between different focus conditions without adverse effects on performance.

For instance a recent publication [98] investigated sprint acceleration in two groups of participants which varied in their skill and experience with this task - specifically, soccer players versus track sprinters. The former group (soccer players) showed the expected outcome: 10m sprint times in the internal focus condition were on average 0.02s slower than external focus or control condition.

Conversely, the track sprinters on average performed the same in the internal focus and control condition; and the average 10m sprint times were actually slightly slower under the external focus condition, albeit this did not reach statistical significance.

Such findings raise questions over whether we should be applying the same rules and conclusions when we dealing with athletes, who by definition possess a high degree of skill and familiarity with the particular movement.

RELATING ATTENTION TO THE TASK...

Aside from skill level, the nature of the task is another factor that might conceivably impact on where the performer should steer their attention.

An illustrative example comes from an investigation [99] that employed a golf pitch shot in high-skill (average golf handicap of 4) and low-skill golfers (mean handicap of 26). For those not familiar with golf, a pitch shot involves lofting the ball in the air to land onto the green as close to the target as possible. In this study, the opposite finding was reported to the sprint acceleration study cited above – adopting an external focus on the target produced better performance in high-skill golfers.

However, perhaps more interesting was that an internal focus of attention (concentrating on the form and force of the swing of the golf club) produced superior performance outcome in the low-skill group. This should raise some doubts over the 'internal focus BAD; external focus GOOD' narrative.

Upon closer inspection, it seems that the story when it comes to locus of attention is not a simple one, and the nature of sports skill or task is an important consideration.

CONSIDERING CONTEXT...

On a similar note, it seems important to consider context in relation to the activity being performed. In the examples so far the sole emphasis has been execution of a complex motor skill. Let us consider how the story might change when the focus switches from skilled execution to endurance. How might locus of attention impact upon the perception of exertion, for instance?

One of the cognitive strategies to modulate perceived exertion is by redirecting locus of attention when engaging in endurance activity. For instance, what researchers describe as an 'associative focus' would be directed towards internal physiological processes, such as breathing rate, heart rate etc. Conversely, a 'dissociative focus' would be directed external to the body, and unrelated to the task of running.

As we might expect, perceived exertion among novice runners tends to be higher with an associative focus, such as attending to sensations of feeling breathless. In contrast, a dissociative focus - for instance concentrating on the scenery - essentially distracts them from the discomfort, and as a result perceived exertion is reduced [100].

Once again, this pattern does not hold true in different populations however. Specifically, the same phenomenon is not observed with endurance runners, who are better able to attend to internal physiological processes and related sensations in a positive way to monitor and modulate output. In fact, endurance runners who employ an associative (internal) focus are reportedly able to maintain higher output (faster running pace) during a race.

Focus of attention during endurance activities can also be directed towards the mechanics of the movement (internal) or outcomes of the movement (external). Interestingly, preliminary evidence [101] suggests that each of these strategies can be employed successfully by different individuals as a way to optimise economy and efficiency, for example when running.

GETTING SPECIFIC ON LOCUS...

As with the instructions provided, the specific aspect or location of the internal or external focus of attention employed is a critical factor that we can expect to affect outcomes and findings of investigations on the topic.

An illustrative example is a study [102] comparing two different internal focus conditions during a golf putting task. There was a contrast in performance outcomes between the two different 'internal focus' conditions according to the specific bodily location where attention was directed. When the internal focus was directed towards a more directly relevant anatomical location in relation to the putting task (hands and elbows) accuracy over the longer putting distance was improved in the novice subjects.

The importance of the specifics of the locus of attention also applies to external focus of attention. For instance, a study of basketball shooting demonstrated external focus of attention trained on the ball served to disrupt shooting performance [103].

The mechanism for the effects observed related to the 'quiet eye' phenomenon, concerning the stability of gaze or fixed visual focus during task execution. Longer 'quiet eye' duration is associated with superior targeting and shooting performance.

Focussing attention on the ball during the shooting task might be expected to cause visual tracking to be unstable, rather than a fixed point of focus. Employing a different external focus fixed on the target (i.e. a stable location such as the basket, rim or backboard) might therefore be more beneficial to shooting performance, as it likely to encourage more stable gaze and longer quiet eye duration.

Interestingly, similar findings were nevertheless noted in a dart throwing study [104], despite instructions to maintain a visual focus on a fixed target (bull's eye) on the dart board. Quiet eye duration in the novice study participants were longer with an internal focus on the throwing arm, whilst keeping their vision fixed on the bull's eye. Despite the same instruction to keep their visual focus on the bull's eye, quiet eye duration was shorter in the external focus condition when participants directed their mental attention on the dart.

TRAINING VERSUS PERFORMING...

Another aspect of attentional focus is that what is desirable in relation to intended outcomes will differ for an athlete in training versus performing in competition.

In the training scenario, the objective is often honing or refining a particular aspect of skill execution. By definition this is likely to require internal focus of attention towards the relevant aspect of the sports skill the coach and athlete are seeking to modify [105]. Unconscious control and 'automaticity' of skill execution might be beneficial in the competition realm. However, these same traits represent a major barrier when the goal is remodelling or refining technical skill or modifying learned coordination patterns.

The few researchers to consider attention in relation to modifying and enhancing skill execution in experienced performers refer to concepts from other realms [105]. In particular, one important consideration is what has been variously termed somatic awareness, body consciousness, and 'somaesthetic perception'. We will consider these aspects and how they relate to honing and refining movement skills in the next section.

Conversely, when it comes to performing in competition the objective is more about delivering execution of well-practiced skills, and managing the pressure of the performance environment. Here the priority switches to avoiding attention becoming distracted and minimising potential disruption to movement skill execution.

In turn this leads us to two types of coping strategies or countermeasures. The first strategy is to avoid potential disruption to the execution or 'automaticity' of the skill. The second coping strategy is to guard against distraction due to the effects of anxiety. We will explore these strategies and how they relate to locus of attention in a later section.

BODY AWARENESS...

In a previous chapter we described body awareness as a pillar of athleticism. Developing sensitivity and specificity with respect to the ability to detect, manipulate and modify aspects of posture and motor control and coordination of limbs and bodily segments is clearly beneficial when we are seeking to correct or hone a particular aspect of a well-learned complex motor skill.

Inwardly directed attention is a central tenet of mindful practice employed to develop body awareness. Likewise, a cornerstone of the process of technical practice is progressively developing the athlete's 'feel' for the movement, their ability to detect errors in coordination and timing, and the facility to self-correct and refine movements. After the athlete performs a repetition of a technical skill invariably the first thing I ask is 'how did that feel?'.

Each of the processes described requires a highly attuned awareness of the athlete's own body and the movement itself. What we are describing here is a type of internal focus of attention.

It is clear that the ability to adapt, correct and refine technical execution is contingent upon an element of internal focus of attention, and this should be a consistent feature of practice and training.

AWARENESS VERSUS CONSCIOUS CONTROL...

There has been a tendency for the research on the topic to treat internal focus of attention as synonymous with 'conscious control'. This is particularly the case when the internal focus of attention condition refers directly to particular aspects of the mechanics of the action.

Authors on the topic rarely seem to consider the possibility that a performer could conceivably direct their attention or awareness towards a body part or aspect of the movement without attempting to consciously control the coordination of the movement itself. Some researchers do make a distinction between 'explicit monitoring' and conscious control. However, even this term implies cognitive noise during skill execution, rather than simply being aware.

Attention is slippery and hard to pin down solely by observing the performer. It might be possible to monitor overt attention, such as where the athlete's gaze is directed or eye tracking. However, covert attention cannot be assessed or manipulated so easily; these are processes that occur in the athlete's own head.

Referring to the 'quiet eye' phenomenon once more, it is altogether possible that an athlete could consciously maintain a stable gaze on a fixed visual target, whilst directing awareness towards an internal focus in relation to the body and/or aspect of the mechanics of the movement.

Equally, if we return to the concept of body awareness, it is also conceivable that an athlete might maintain a level of body awareness even as they direct their focus of attention towards the outcome or goal of the movement and attend to relevant information in the environment.

More simply, an internal locus of attention does not necessarily need to be to the exclusion of external focus, and vice versa. It is entirely conceivable that skilled performers in particular will possess the attentional capacity to maintain both internal and external foci simultaneously.

ACCOUNTING FOR PREFERRED OR ACCUSTOMED FOCUS...

A notable finding reported by a number of studies is that when the task is carried out under a neutral condition (i.e. no attentional cues provided) there is a fairly equally distribution of participants who subsequently report using an internal focus versus external focus of attention.

Clearly a variety of strategies may be employed successfully. These observations also raise the interesting possibility that what constitutes the most appropriate locus of attention may depend on the individual. Perhaps we should therefore allow the individual the freedom to self-select their locus of attention, based on natural inclination and preference.

In relation to this, an important finding of research investigations is that what locus of attention is optimal (or sub-optimal) depends on what the individual is familiar with or accustomed to using. Decrements in performance are most consistently observed under 'forced' conditions where the participant is instructed to employ the alternate 'unfamiliar' focus condition that they are not accustomed to [106].

CONSIDERING INDIVIDUAL DISPOSITION...

Studies suggest that the effects of focus of attention manipulations may be greater under pressure conditions. It is also possible this will have greater impact on certain individuals who differ in 'trait anxiety', or disposition to experience anxiety in response to a perceived threat or daunting situation. It is demonstrated that some performers are more prone to 'reinvestment' under pressure, and the adverse performance effects of anxiety (often termed 'choking').

One study [107] demonstrated that those scoring high on the 'reinvestment scale' can be more susceptible to reinvesting conscious control in response to an internal focus condition that focussed undue attention on a particular facet of the task. HOWEVER, this was not the case when they employed an alternative internal focus on a process goal that they were able to self-select.

Therefore whilst care must be taken when dealing with individuals who are more prone to anxiety and score higher on the 'reinvestment scale', if the correct internal focus or process goal is employed these problems may be avoided.

Individual athletes also sit on different points on the introversion vs extroversion continuum. Those who identify as introvert by definition will have a greater tendency to look inwards (introspection). It follows that for these individuals there might be a greater need to escape their own heads, as this will be default setting. Conceivably, encouraging introvert-type athletes towards an external focus of attention might be beneficial from this viewpoint. Equally there are also other coping strategies that might be employed.

COPING STRATEGIES AND COUNTERMEASURES...

Under pressure conditions it is documented [108] that there is a tendency to focus more inwardly, termed 'self-focused attention'. In a competition scenario, this makes for a compelling argument that we should steer athletes' attention towards an external focus to combat the inclination to 'reinvest' conscious control.

Equally, if the athlete is able to control their attention and associated movement behaviour under pressure, so that their normal locus of attention and process does not differ from what is customary to perform successfully in training, then this is unlikely to be an issue.

A major source of distraction in a pressure environment can be anxious thoughts, including self-talk and imagining scenarios or consequences.

Once again, adopting an external focus of attention is often advocated as an effective countermeasure. This offers a way to steer the performer's attention and awareness away from anxious thoughts and feelings; in essence, distracting them from potential internal distractions. External focus of attention can also be helpful to ensure the performer attends to relevant information in the competition environment amidst their anxiety.

There are however a range of other mental tools and coping strategies performers might use. One example is 'quiet eye' training, which demonstrates beneficial effects on performance under pressure. Fundamentally, it is important to recognise that the distraction comes from the anxious thoughts and associated physical sensations, rather than an internal focus of attention per se.

For instance, just as controlling gaze is beneficial, the performer might equally direct their focus towards the process (i.e. internal focus) as a means to stay in the moment and keep from being distracted by anxious thoughts and mental projections. Allowing the athlete to select an appropriate process focus appears equally beneficial for performance under pressure, regardless of propensity for reinvestment and 'choking'.

MOVING BEYOND THE DOMINANT NARRATIVE...

In summary, the question of where to direct athletes' attention, and what cues to employ, is clearly more complex than the 'internal focus BAD; external focus GOOD' message that is currently being espoused to coaches and practitioners in the field.

As always, 'it depends'. It depends on what population we are dealing with (for instance, novices versus skilled performers). It depends on task and context. It depends on whether we are speaking about training or competition. And it depends on the individual, and their natural inclination and disposition.

On the broader question of how best to instruct and direct athletes, a few major themes emerge.

The first key theme is that we must be considered and concise in what instruction we provide. Whether we are dealing in external or internal cues, less is more. The critical objective is providing the salient information and appropriate guidance whilst avoiding bombarding the athlete with extraneous noise and tying them in knots. The coach can be the worst source of distraction and misdirection when learning a skill.

The second take-home message is that details and specifics matter. Particularly when thinking about internal cues, precisely where the athlete's attention is directed with respect to bodily location, and what specific facet of the skill is highlighted, are decisive to the outcome. This critical detail is lost in the facile internal versus external focus debates.

Finally, each of these aspects of attention and instruction will be highly specific to the individual. Knowing the athlete is key to discovering the approach that works best for them. Arriving at the best approach to guiding learning, and where and how to direct attention, will be a journey of exploring different cues and methods, supported by an ongoing process of reflecting and refining

'Emotional Control' is a Superpower for Athletes

Traits such as 'resilience' and 'mental toughness' are frequently referred to in elite sport. Coping with the challenges of competing at elite level and the associated pressures is clearly critical for athletes. However, we also need to consider how the athlete manages the challenges that exist in their life outside of the sporting arena. The athlete's psychological state and emotional wellbeing has a profound bearing on how they are able to function in their sport. There is a growing realisation of the impact of non-training stressors in the context of planning and periodisation. Recent insights from research investigations show that how the athlete appraises a situation has a major bearing on how they anticipate and experience these events, and the physiological and emotional responses that result. These perspectives indicate the importance of emotional intelligence and emotion regulation for athletes. As we will explore in this chapter, an athlete's ability to exercise control in how they appraise events and regulate emotional responses are critical factors that will impact upon their wellbeing, and in turn their ability to handle challenges and cope with the stresses of training and competing.

PERCEPTION SHAPES EMOTION…

"Our emotional state is largely determined by what we attend to…"

— Daniel Kahneman

Our immediate environment has a major bearing on our emotional state. In the context of sport, this includes both the sporting domain and the athlete's personal life. The people we surround ourselves with, and our interactions with those we encounter in our day to day environment have a profound effect on our emotional state and general wellbeing.

We are beginning to understand how pervasive the effects of others' behaviour are on our emotional and physiological state. The phenomenon of 'stress contagion' and its physiological mechanisms have received recent investigation [109]. Generally emotional intelligence is viewed as a very positive trait, as this enables us to negotiate social interactions better and allows for more meaningful relationships. Interestingly in this instance, more empathetic individuals (empathy being highly associated with emotional intelligence) appear to be more susceptible to being affected by the behaviour and 'emotional expression' of others [109].

What we focus our attention on, with respect to day-to-day events and interactions, similarly serves to shape our mood. By extension, we are particularly influenced by what we dwell on after the event. These 'ruminations' following a given event or troubling interaction have a major bearing on our state. Moreover, these effects persist long after the event itself; indeed for as long as we ruminate upon them.

EMOTION SHAPES PERCEPTION…

Conversely, our mood also colours how we see the world. Both temperament and acute emotional state can profoundly influence how we perceive our environment [110]. Particularly pertinent to sport is that this extends to how we perceive opportunities for action within our environment. For instance, it has been demonstrated that an individual's perception of height and distance can be influenced by their emotional state at that given time [111].

Two key elements in relation to perception are psychological arousal and emotional state. The term 'emotional valence' has been employed to differentiate between positive and negative mood states [112]. Individual temperament also comes into play, as this will influence both how prone we are to negative emotions, and also helps to determine our default response to arousal.

Negative affect is a blanket term used for emotional states that we consider to be negative, 'toxic', or debilitating. Examples of emotional states of negative affect include anxiety and depression. Anger is often included under this umbrella; however investigations indicate that anger does not entirely fit the profile from a neurobiological viewpoint [113].

The inter-relationship between emotional state and perception may have implications for direct perception and how we perceive the action opportunities of objects and features of the movement landscape [111]. For instance, when we are in a negative emotional state it is conceivable that this may influence what we perceive to be possible.

In this way, emotional state can impact our behaviour in a sporting context, due to the coupling between perception-action. In essence, our state influences our perception of what is possible or viable, and in turn this is reflected in the actions we take as a result.

Emotion can affect perception and thereby movement behaviour in other ways. Mood state has been implicated in where we direct our visual attention [110]. When we are troubled we are often distracted. In this state we are more susceptible to attending to irrelevant stimuli and failing to attend to relevant stimuli.

Finally, there is some evidence that negative affect or mood state may impact our capacity for learning. Whilst this is not a consistent finding, one study that manipulated mood state indicated that participants in the negative affect condition showed poorer scores for implicit learning on the serial reaction task employed [114].

THE PERVASIVE EFFECTS OF 'AFFECT'…

It is important to recognise that emotion is a 'psycho-physiological' phenomenon [109]. In simple terms, our psychological and physiological state are closely inter-related. Our mood state affects our physiology, including our physiological response under different conditions. For instance, the acute state of negative affect (emotions such as anxiety) are related to stress hormone responses [113].

Personality traits have a bearing on our emotional state and thereby our physiological state. The effects associated with 'trait negative affect' therefore also include altered autonomic nervous system function. Those who self-reported being prone to anxiety and depression showed altered cardiac autonomic function, based on heart rate variability measures [113].

Moving beyond personality traits, events in an individual's life can be a source of acute (short-term) stress. Operating under conditions of elevated life stress impairs an athlete's ability to recover from training [115]. Associated measures of muscle function, such as force output, are also depressed during the recovery period in those reporting higher scores for life stress [116].

If these circumstances persist, and the athlete is operating under a chronic state of stress, the added strain not only impact their ability to perform during training and competition, and recover in between, but will also affect their health. Periods of elevated life stress are reflected in epidemics of illness and injury among athlete. For instance, a study of student athletes demonstrated huge spikes in rates of illness and injury during periods of high academic stress (exam time) [117].

Avoiding illness and injury are clearly critical to enable consistent participation in training. Avoiding enforced absences in training due to illness and injury is demonstrated to be a primary factor that differentiates those who are able to achieve their performance goals [35].

Given these findings it is unsurprising that negative emotional states are viewed as toxic to the individual. Negative affect has even been identified as a potential factor in the pathophysiology of coronary heart disease.

COMBATING THE TOXICITY...

The literature on 'psychological resilience' in relation to sports performers identifies the role of 'mental processes and behaviour' [118] in protecting against the potential negative effects of stressors and challenges from a variety of sources in the life of the athlete.

It is important to note here that every athlete brings their own innate characteristics and personality traits. The temperament of each individual is generally considered to be hardwired or 'biologically-driven'. We can consider this the 'default setting' that is unique to the individual. Clearly we need to give consideration to the individual traits of each athlete in our quest to combat the negative 'sequelae' or cascade of physiological effects triggered by life stress and pressures of the training and competition environment.

The task of empowering an athlete to exercise control and counteract the toxic effects of negative affect will therefore differ for each individual. The temperament of the individual provides the context or landscape when seeking to devising strategies and constructing coping mechanisms.

Whilst temperament is innate and drives our 'natural' response to events in an unconscious way, there is nevertheless scope to exercise conscious control over the process.

KNOW THYSELF…

Emotional intelligence is distinct from other forms of intelligence. Individuals differ widely in emotional intelligence, in a way that is independent of other metrics of intelligence. An individual with a high IQ can exhibit low emotional intelligence, and vice versa. In essence, emotional intelligence describes the degree to which we are able to make best use of our emotions [119]. A related index of emotional intelligence is the propensity to behave in a way that is responsive and appropriate to the emotions of others.

A frank and honest appraisal of our personality traits and temperament will allow us to understand our individual 'default setting' and gain insights into our hardwired responses so that we can use our emotions to better effect. Self-awareness is critical to being able to detect our own emotional state at a given time and emotional responses to events in the moment. Without the necessary self-awareness the task of understanding our emotional state and reflecting upon how we react to events and stimuli clearly becomes very difficult.

External input can be very helpful in this process, and indeed may be necessary. Nevertheless, the individual must drive the initiative. Indeed, to be most receptive the individual should actively seek out external input. The most value will come from trusted sources who know the individual well, and are able to be unflinching in providing a frank and honest perspective. In turn, it is incumbent upon the individual to take the feedback provided on board.

Armed with an awareness of our predisposition and how we are likely to react in a given situation, we can devise strategies and countermeasures to help self-regulate our responses in real-time.

RECOGNISING CHOICE…

Rather than passively accepting that we are at the mercy of our environment and other people, it is important to recognise the element of choice. Whilst we must operate under certain constraints, it is within our power to exercise some degree of choice in where we spend our time and with whom.

"You cannot change those around you… but you can change those you choose to be around"

— Anon

Moreover, it is absolutely in our power to exercise voluntary control over the situations we involve ourselves in, what we choose to attend to, and what we invest our time and mental resources ruminating upon.

VOLUNTARY REGULATION OF EMOTIONAL RESPONSE...

Investing in becoming more self-aware provides the opportunity to exercise some voluntary control over our emotional responses. Understanding that we may be prone to a particular state and predisposed to react in a certain way might allow us to modify or modulate our dominant response, and cultivate 'non-dominant' responses [120]. In the literature this voluntary and deliberate regulation is sometimes termed 'effortful control'.

On a fundamental level this is not about suppressing our emotions or changing who we are. Rather, it is a question of accepting and better understanding ourselves in order to both anticipate and recognise hardwired emotional reactions as they occur. In essence, we are working with our emotions, rather than simply being a slave to our involuntary responses.

If we can acknowledge emotional states that do not serve us well we can mitigate the impact, and give ourselves the option of modulating our emotional reaction and behaviours when there is a need to do so. We can manifest emotional regulation in a variety of ways, including altering the intensity of our emotional response to a situation, the time-course, and how we experience the emotional response.

Circling back, being self-aware of our emotional state is clearly paramount, as this will influence how we are predisposed to reacting to certain events or external stimuli. Exercising voluntary regulation is therefore a dynamic task with shifting constraints that are shaped by our emotional state at any given time.

Exercising self-awareness and practising self-reflection are therefore integral to developing the capability to regulate and modify our involuntary responses over time. Inevitably this will be an ongoing process. There will be lessons to take from the different challenges and circumstances we encounter on the journey.

The ongoing process and reflective practice are also likely to benefit from outside guidance and periodic external input. This may be in the form of debriefs or reviews at appropriate intervals with a coach, a mentor, or perhaps somebody from our life beyond sport.

MANAGING EMOTIONAL TRIGGERS...

With the benefit of experience and reflection we can gain important insights into situations and scenarios that trigger us in a negative way. More importantly we can put this information to work and take pre-emptive action.

One route to better managing situations to mitigate the emotional impact is to alter our cognition surrounding the event. In the literature this strategy is termed 'cognitive change' [121].

> "Cognitive change... changing the way we think in order to change the way we feel"
>
> — Pena-Sarrionandia and colleagues, 2015 [119]

In essence, we can appraise the scenario in a different way to shift our perception, and thereby alter the emotional response that occurs as a result. Simply adopting a different and perhaps more objective or 'rational' perspective can take some of the emotional sting out of how we anticipate and experience the same event.

REGULATING RUMINATION AFTER THE EVENT...

Whilst we can regulate our initial emotional response somewhat, some type of reaction is entirely natural, and this not something we should be looking to eliminate entirely. What we can exercise some control over is our cognitive processing after the event.

Ruminating or dwelling on what has occurred can serve to prolong the effect on our emotional state. As such, the tendency to ruminate is strongly linked to the pathophysiological responses observed among individuals [121]. How we choose to deal with what has occurred therefore has a major bearing on our emotional state during the (extended) period following the original inciting event.

From this viewpoint it appears critical to process events in a timely manner, or find a way to let it go, in order to minimise the lingering effect on our emotional state in the period that follows. This cognitive processing might involve rationalising what has occurred, to achieve some separation between our emotional response and the event itself. Metaphorically stepping away in our view of the event allows the necessary perspective to enable us to deal with what has occurred and move past it.

Communicating and confiding what has occurred is likely to be beneficial to avoid internalising and ruminating upon what has occurred in a way that foments further negative emotion. Accordingly, social support is identified as an important protective factor from a resilience viewpoint, or more specifically the athlete's perception of what social support is available to them [118]. Sharing what has occurred with others can also assist the athlete in working through what has occurred, take any lessons, and decide on any further action to take to resolve any ongoing issues moving forward.

Finally, there is some preliminary evidence that practising 'mindfulness' can reduce individuals' tendency for rumination [122].

PRACTISING MINDFULNESS...

Whilst mindfulness has become a popular term in sport, most often it is vague and poorly defined. The definition taken from the study cited previously is: "present-centred non-judgemental awareness of internal and external stimuli where an individual attends to all these events on a moment-to-moment basis without trying to control, change or avoid any of these internal experiences" [122].

Whilst the wording is likely to elicit a certain amount of eye-rolling from athletes and coaches, the above definition is somewhat useful for identifying some key tenets that can help inform how we might employ mindfulness in practice.

The first key point of this practice is that the athlete strives to maintain their attention on the present, rather than ruminating on what has gone before, or contemplating what might happen in the future. What follows from this is that the athlete attends to their immediate environment, as well as their thoughts and feelings in the present moment. The latter speaks to the awareness of self and present emotional state that we have spoken about previously.

The final salient points in the definition of mindfulness in practice are that the individuals accepts what is occurring, and attends to it without judgement. Of all the elements, the latter is perhaps the most likely to be questioned and is surely the most challenging to achieve in practice. Whilst it may not be entirely achievable, striving to suspend judgement can nevertheless be viewed as a noble endeavour.

EGO-RESILIENCY...

Another aspect of how we process negative outcomes or events is ego-resiliency. Ego-resiliency has been conceptualised as an adaptive 'higher-order' skill or executive function, akin to problem solving [120]. In essence, resiliency comprises flexible coping and regulation strategies that evolve as we reflect on experiences and refine our approach over time.

In particular, ego-resiliency is pertinent to how we are able to respond to and bounce back from negative events, and emotional 'legacy effects' that follow adverse outcomes within the sporting arena.

On a deeper level, ego resiliency leads us into the realms of self-concept. As such, this requires us to explore and tackle some issues from a more 'humanistic' perspective [123]. Good coaches and practitioners understand the value and importance of relating to the athlete as a human beyond the confines of the sport. Equally it is critical that the athlete is able to do the same in relation to themselves.

If an athlete cannot separate their self-concept from their goals and identity within the sport then this clearly raises the stakes exponentially. Frequently we try to reassure the athlete by telling them it is not life and death. We need to consider that if their whole concept of self is essentially at stake then to the athlete themselves it can easily seem like a life and death matter.

Objectively, without any separation between self-concept and sport the life of the athlete can be a fragile existence. With the athlete so precariously balanced on such an uncertain foundation this existence can easily become untenable, or certainly only sustainable at great emotional cost to the individual.

We must help athletes to step away and 'zoom out' to gain a higher vantage point and a wider perspective on the world. We should also encourage them to invest in their life outside sport, so that they can find validation beyond the sporting realm.

NEVER SATISFIED...

Athletes and coaches we are often in an almost perpetual state being dissatisfied, or rather not entirely satisfied with our present level or a particular outcome. How we are disposed towards these events and the mood that the experience elicits is largely defined by our perception and expectations.

It is fine to want more, and to be driven to do better; indeed, this is one of the attributes that differentiates the elite performer. The question is more how we view this lack of total satisfaction, and our insatiable hunger to achieve.

Once more this comes down to mind-set and perspective. One option is to have negative feelings or associations with not being satisfied. Equally, it is possible to experience the same situation in a positive way, to spur us ever onwards in the knowledge that there is always more and new goals to strive for.

GIVING FULL ATTENTION TO THE GOOD STUFF...

It is not necessarily a bad thing that we are never 100% satisfied with the outcome. Nevertheless, it does make it all the more important that the athlete is able to take the small wins in the day to day process.

One reason that entitlement is so toxic is that the individual derives very little pleasure from their successes in training and competition. After all, they are simply getting what they feel is their due and consider to be theirs by right. It is the curse of entitlement that these individuals will also feel resentful in every other instance.

From this viewpoint, it is valuable to consciously direct our attention to the positive facets of our environment. We should steer our awareness and give full consideration to the elements in our existence that give us cause to feel positive and content.

Gratitude is rightly increasingly identified as a powerful tool in relation to positive affect and our sense of wellbeing. Actively giving consideration to how blessed and fortunate we are can have a profound effect on our emotional state and general wellbeing. In turn, negative emotions such as resentment do not readily coexist with gratitude. It is hard to feel bitter or resentful when reminding ourselves what we have to feel grateful for.

STRESS TESTING...

In the heat of battle our attention is likely to be diverted and our working capacity can be overwhelmed. In this scenario we are likely to revert back to our default setting, and in the absence of any conscious regulation our 'unedited' hardwired responses may once more come to the fore.

Conditions of pressure and heightened challenge also offer the opportunity to stress test these adaptive mental skills. Exposure to pressure conditions is therefore an important part of honing these coping skills, developing resilience, and becoming better able to respond to setbacks.

Once again, how we appraise the situation is important here. We can strive to alter how we anticipate and deal with the prospect of pressure situations where there is the possibility of failing. Over time, we can shift from appraising this prospect as threatening and negative to a new perspective, whereby we view it as an opportunity to stress test and develop our coping skills and capabilities under performance conditions.

Ultimately, this process of reappraisal offers a means for the athlete to take back control. This newfound sense of control allows a change in how they entertain pressure situations, so that rather than avoiding the 'threat', the athlete eventually comes to invite and actively seek out these opportunities, as they strive to develop their mental skills and work towards a desired outcome.

Section Three – Managing Self

A Self-Regulated Learning Path to More Productive Preparation

A thletes and coaches across all sports incessantly speak about the importance of 'focussing on the process', and process goals. As coaches and practitioners we are likewise ever mindful of scheduling constraints and the need to make best use of the finite time permitted to prepare our athletes. In previous chapters we have spoken about the importance of mobilising mental resources, and the critical role of athletes' perception in relation to training responses. Here we will venture into the realms of teaching and learning, in order to make meaningful use of the notion of 'process focus' in the context of sport. In our quest for more purposeful training we will explore the concept of self-regulated learning', and outline how these principles might be applied to the process and the practice of preparing athletes.

Meta-Learning: the state of 'being aware of and taking control of one's own learning'

— John Biggs

LEARNING HOW TO LEARN EFFECTIVELY...

The concept of 'meta-learning' refers to the processes that govern and underpin the learning process. These principles apply across different domains. Critical elements include the learner's awareness of their own learning process, consideration of how best to approach learning a task or topic, and the ongoing 'metacognitive' processes of selecting, reviewing and refining the strategy employed over time.

In the present era of connectivity and incessant distractions from mobile technology and social media, authors in the field of education identify that young people increasingly struggle to develop study skills and the ability to self-regulate their learning. These observations from a scholastic realm equally apply to sport and athletic preparation.

Coaching has many parallels to teaching. It is no coincidence that historically many elite coaches and practitioners have come from a teaching background. For any coach or practitioner, I would contend that adopting a teaching perspective is entirely more useful than taking a 'service industry' viewpoint, as is becoming increasingly common in the field.

On a fundamental level, in the training environment we are challenging the athlete to learn and adapt. As outlined in a previous chapter, we can conceptualise training as a problem-solving exercise. We also spoke in the previous section about the power of mobilising mental resources and how this can impact the quality of training input and the adaptation that ensues.

If we acknowledge that it is important to learn how to learn more effectively, in a sporting context it is equally critical for an athlete to learn how to train more productively.

EVIDENCE OF A DIFFERENT APPROACH IN SUCCESSFUL ATHLETES...

Investigations of 'talented' athletes in different sports indicate that an apparent point of difference with more successful performers is the level of planning and effort they invest in their approach to training and practice.

In particular, critical elements of 'self-regulation' simply involves the athlete being self-directed and proactive in their approach to their own development. The degree to which athletes take responsibility for their own learning and practice can be demonstrated in their behaviours both during and outside of sessions.

Accordingly these 'self-regulatory' behaviours and cognitive processes that underpin training seem to be part of what differentiates successful performers in different sports. For instance, preliminary evidence [124] indicates that part of what separates elite and non-elite team sports players is the level of self-awareness of their own areas of strength and weakness. Clearly what is also crucial is how the athlete makes use of this knowledge.

A key point of difference noted in the previous study is the level of effort and attention athletes habitually invest during training sessions [124]. Another important factor that has been identified is the level of forethought the athlete brings to their practice [125].

Self-directed learning and self-regulatory practices appear to be particularly critical in certain sports. Notably, self-regulatory learning behaviours are reportedly more prevalent among athletes in individual sports [126].

A DELIBERATE APPROACH TO PRACTICE...

Long term athlete development models refer to the 'learn to train' phase as an integral part of the developmental process. Yet beyond this acknowledgement, it is very rare that athletes are actually provided with any tangible direction on how they might learn to train more effectively.

For the most part, athletes do not customarily give any real consideration to their approach to the training process, and what strategies they might employ to make best use of these opportunities to develop.

The concept of self-regulated learning concerns the individual's control and regulation of their own learning behaviour, including their feelings towards the endeavour, the cognitive processes they employ during learning, and their motivation in pursuing identified objectives. Notable authors in the field, such as Barry J. Zimmerman [125], have pioneered the application of concepts of 'self-regulated learning' to motor learning in the context of sport, particularly with young athletes.

By definition, engaging in deliberate practice is dependent upon the individual having the capacity to summon the motivation and mental faculties required to immerse themselves in what is a highly effortful pursuit [127].

Self-regulated learning in the context of deliberate practice provides an explanation for what differentiates quality of practice and discriminates individual differences in outcomes and acquisition of expertise [128]. The athlete's propensity for self-regulated learning will allow them to optimise their practice, so that a greater proportion of the hours of practice they engage in are of high quality.

SELF-REGULATION AND ATHLETE DEVELOPMENT...

From a group of individuals engaging in practice, those who are more invested, focussed, and proficient from a self-regulated learning viewpoint are likely to show superior development over time. Self-regulated learning, and the elements which underpin it, are therefore immerging as critical factors for long-term success from an athlete development viewpoint [128].

In this chapter, we will extend the application of 'self-regulated learning' principles to all facets of physical and athletic preparation. Just as many in the field extol the virtues of 'deliberate practice', by extension it is also beneficial to be deliberate in our approach to training.

Young athletes in particular are likely to require additional guidance in this area. In essence, we need to help provide them with the necessary tools if we want them to be focussed, deliberate and systematic in their approach to their preparation.

As we explore in the next section, practices that place the athlete in the centre of the training process are crucial to supporting and preserving intrinsic motivation in the pursuit.

THE ROLE OF THE ATHLETE IN THE TRAINING PROCESS...

A feature of modern elite and professional sport is a preoccupation with 'high performance teams' as comprising an extensive array of specialist support staff. In the drive to provide comprehensive specialist support what can be lost is the role of the athlete in directing and regulating their own practice and preparation.

We generally assume that the athlete is invested in becoming better. However, even for an athlete who is fully engaged, in many instances they can nevertheless find their role in the daily training process becomes somewhat passive. Professional team settings or high performance systems can operate in such a way that responsibility for the day-to-day process is unwittingly delegated to the respective member of the support staff, so that the onus is taken away from the athlete.

Likewise, in a commercial setting, where the athlete (or parent) is paying for coaching services, there can also be a 'transactional mind-set' – i.e. 'it is your job to make me better'. This not only abdicates responsibility, but also renders it very difficult to hold the athlete accountable to the process or the outcome.

Fundamentally, the intention the athlete brings to their training, and the attention and mental effort they invest each time they train, are critical to the outcome. By definition the athlete is an active player in the process; their role and contribution must be continually emphasised.

Indeed, self-regulated learning implies that the athlete is not only an active player, but is proactive in the process. Over time the athlete should assume a more active role in driving their own preparation. The culture of the team and the daily training environment must facilitate this.

'THE GRIND': PRACTICE HOURS VERSUS YIELD...

In the media (and social media) a worrisome trend is that we increasingly hear athletes and even coaches refer to 'the grind'. This is a problem. Promoting the notion of grinding through hours of practice or training in a mindless manner is entirely unhelpful.

It is crucial that we recognise that hours of practice logged by an athlete are not equal in quality or yield. When it comes to acquiring and honing skilled performance, a single hour of 'deep' mindful practice will yield far greater results than multiple hours of mindless repetition.

In the same way we should give greater consideration to the quality of all aspects of physical and athletic preparation undertaken by an athlete. Training exposure alone does not equate to outcome. It is not sufficient to merely show and go through the motions.

Attendance is clearly an important starting point; showing up provides the athlete the opportunity to improve and develop. However, taking advantage of the opportunity afforded when the athlete comes to training is contingent on what mental resources they invest each day.

THE QUEST FOR MINDFUL PRACTICE...

Connecting mind and body is the holy grail when it comes to athletic preparation. Along with time, attention represents a precious and increasingly scarce resource.

Being 'mindful' first requires the athlete to exercise some awareness of their own process, and give consideration to how they approach their preparation. These are critical pillars of self-regulation, and yet are often overlooked.

If you ask an aspiring athlete whether they have given any thought to how they approach their skill practice, it is entirely possible that this has never occurred to them. I would venture that the likelihood is even less if you were to ask whether they have given any serious thought to how they approach their physical preparation.

As we have spoken about in a previous chapter, the intention that the athlete brings to their practice and training is crucial to the outcome. Arguably this begins even before the training session commences. The athlete should be clear in their aims and objectives from the moment that they arrive at the training facility; and if not, they should take the time to 'dial in' before beginning the session.

CRITICAL PARTS OF THE PROCESS BEHIND THE PROCESS...

Borrowing once again from the self-regulated learning literature, we can identify four major pillars for self-directed preparation practices. These pillars are goal setting, evaluation, monitoring, and reflection.

#1 DEFINE ASPIRATIONS, AIMS, AND OBJECTIVES...

Goal-setting is a critical process whereby the athlete sets their intention in relation to skill acquisition and physical development. From the outset the athlete must identify their long-term aspirations, medium-term aims or outcomes, and objectives they are working towards in the short-term.

Clearly, setting goals is a good way to provide direction. Beyond this, having some clearly defined aims and outcomes also provides something to hold the athlete accountable to. The athlete's aims and objectives will naturally evolve over time, and so should be reviewed periodically and updated as necessary.

Each day the athlete should be prompted to remind themselves why they are there, what they are working towards, and the person they want to be. In this way the imagined future version of themselves that they aspire to be serves as both a 'virtual' role model and the standard that they hold themselves to on a day-to-day basis.

#2 SELF-EVALUATION...

To be deliberate and systematic in their approach requires the athlete to be aware and give consideration to their role in the process. Self-awareness is not only the starting point, but is also integral to each step of the process that follows.

A simple questionnaire can be employed to allow the athlete to evaluate their current status and rate themselves on different aspects. This provides be the starting point for further discussions during the review process. An example is provided in the appendix that follows the final chapter.

#3 ONGOING MONITORING...

Just as self-awareness is the foundation, self-monitoring is a critical practice that underpins self-regulated learning and a self-directed approach to athletic preparation. Self-recording is the formal process for this.

In a recent conversation with Ben Rosenblatt he made a compelling argument for putting the onus back on the athlete, particularly with respect to daily monitoring practices.

Clearly it is beneficial for the athlete to keep a record of their training, and log the sets and repetitions completed. It is also in the athlete's interests to be diligent in completing the daily monitoring tools they employ (e.g. sleep and wellness measures). Given that these tools are intended for the athlete's benefit, there should be a clear expectation that the athlete should take responsibility for them.

There are important implications here that extend to the athlete's life beyond training facility. Lifestyle factors are critical in supporting training adaptation, and from a health and injury viewpoint. These factors are entirely dependent upon the behaviours and decisions the athlete takes when beyond the reach of the coach or practitioner. Given that it is ultimately incumbent upon the individual, personal responsibility must therefore be emphasised and reinforced as an integral part of the culture of the training environment.

#4 REVIEW AND REFLECTION...

Just as we have spoken about reflective practice as critical for coaches and practitioners, it is equally crucial that athletes exercise reflection. Implementing a practice strategy is of limited value without the facility to evaluate its effectiveness, and to reflect and refine their approach over time.

Dan Pfaff emphasises the importance of the daily debrief as an integral part of the training process. It is important for the athlete to record their own observations on the process as a basis for reflection; the use of a training journal allows the athlete to record any information that is pertinent, including coaching cues that resonated and also their own cognitive strategies. In-depth review and feedback sessions should also be scheduled at regular intervals, usually following the completion of each training block.

In combination these elements provide the framework for the athlete to reflect upon the training process on an ongoing basis. In turn these tools and processes further prompt the athlete to consider how might alter how they approach their training to improve outcomes, and seek any guidance to assist them to do so.

CLOSING REMARKS...

The process behind the process matters. The level of awareness, attention and thought the athlete brings to their preparation are critical factors. It follows that as coaches and practitioners we should give greater consideration to athlete's role in the preparation process.

There are a number of different pillars and processes that can help inform and support how the athlete approaches their training and practice. Just as this is critical for skill practice, the same emphasis should also be applied to how an athlete approaches their physical and athletic preparation.

Mindful 'deep practice' is effortful and requires considerable investment of mental resources. This is much the same with physical preparation. As such, a willingness to invest effort and attention on the part of the athlete is a critical trait and a likely determinant of their future success in the sport. This is particularly the case with individual sports given that self-regulatory learning behaviours appear more prevalent among successful performers in these sports.

Developing the pillars of self-regulated learning behaviours are likely to confer wider benefits. For instance, developing self-awareness and educating the athlete on taking responsibility for their own development are important for their own sake. These are desirable traits, and the disciplines they develop will have positive transfer to the scholastic realm and the athlete's life beyond sport.

Handling Major Competition

Major competition poses unique challenges not only for the athlete, but also the coach and wider support staff. From a logistical viewpoint there are a host of additional factors to manage, but on a more personal level, each member of the team must also manage themselves and how they interact with the athlete. In the crucible of a major competition environment the mettle of all individuals concerned is tested, and every member of staff connected to the athlete has a responsibility. In this chapter we will dig deeper on this topic, and explore ways we can support athletes in handling the pressures to compete at their best on the biggest stage.

It is tempting to think that once the athlete arrives at a major competition much of the work of the coach is essentially done. Certainly this is not a time for excessive external input, introducing a lot of new information, or indeed doing 'work', beyond final touches to prime the athlete and optimise readiness. Nevertheless, the coach still has a critical part to play, and this goes beyond tactical and technical input. Positively influencing the athlete's mental and emotional state, and assisting the athlete in managing the challenges and pressures associated with a major competition environment can be hugely important to the outcome.

It also important to note that these discussions concern not only the sports coach or technical coach but all practitioners involved (physical preparation, physiotherapist etc). Indeed all members of staff attending have a duty of care and some level of coaching responsibility towards the athlete. Moreover, these considerations do not just concern what happens once the athlete arrives at the stadium. Managing the periods leading up to the event, and in the gaps between practices, matches or sessions during the event can be equally critical.

STAFF DUTY OF CARE...

During the crucial phases in the competition calendar the human interaction element of coaching comes to the fore. And once again, when the athlete arrives at major competition every practitioner and staff member in contact with the athlete needs to be aware of this crucial aspect and their responsibilities to the athlete.

From a coach or practitioner viewpoint the approach to the competition and the event itself demands a high level of emotional intelligence. In particular, self-awareness and a high degree of empathy are required of all staff in regular contact with the athlete. The ability to read the athlete and the situation becomes critical in communicating and behaving in a manner that is helpful. All staff must remain mindful that their behaviour is a potential trigger for adding to the stress of the situation.

"Mindfulness applies not only to the coach, but to the athlete and the performance staff. We have had therapists that were awesome on game day, and we have had therapists that were absolute nightmares on game day, because pressure and the distractions at the majors got them away from being mindful and their task."

— Dan Pfaff

The phenomenon of 'stress contagion' is a very real danger, particularly in the crucible of competition [109]. It is the responsibility of all staff members to exercise a high level of awareness and remain vigilant in how they conduct themselves. Indulging the urge to fret is not a luxury anybody can afford. Anxiety is contagious. Stress-signalling behaviour on the part of staff members will inevitably communicate itself to the athlete to some degree, impacting their physiological and emotional state, and adding to the stress of the situation. This 'empathic stress' is particularly likely to be apparent with athletes who are high in empathy [109].

THE PERVERSE LOGIC OF PRE-CAMPS...

One of the great ironies of major competitions, championship games, or play-off series is that athletes are customarily brought into an unfamiliar environment during their final preparations.

I recall Dan Pfaff speaking on the topic during my visit to Altis in late 2015. Dan urged the coaches and practitioners in attendance to avoid national federation 'pre-camps' or holding camps prior to major championships where possible. This is a coach who knows something of coaching at major competitions: Rio 2016 was his 10th Olympic games as a coach, and until London 2017 Dan had attended every athletics world championships since their inception in 1983.

The notion of removing the athlete and coach from their normal working environment to bring them into a pre-camp environment with an entirely different social dynamic and constraints that are not normally present does not make a great deal of sense, particularly in view of the stress and pressures of the competition to come. This practice is all the more nonsensical for individual sports.

Given that the athlete and coach operate (quite successfully) in a completely different way for the other 11+ months of the year, it is baffling that at the most critical time they should be transplanted into an alien environment and have their normal processes disrupted.

The strain of the team hotel environment or athletes' village at a major competition must also be recognised. Athletes and coaches dwell within this 'bubble' for the duration of the event or play-off series. Once again, stipulating that athletes and coaches must stay 'in camp' ahead of the event only adds to the strain, particularly for those who find this environment restricting and somewhat claustrophobic.

This phenomenon can also be observed in other sports. For a championship game or play-offs there are often misguided efforts to make the occasion 'more special' by changing the players' normal routine and preparation environment, and adding superfluous bells and whistles, such as a 'special' match day outfit for the occasion.

STRIVING FOR NORMALCY...

"Leadership is a matter of having people look at you and gain confidence, seeing how you react. If you're in control, they're in control.

— Tom Landry

Given the disruptions and distractions that inevitably accompany major events in the competition calendar, it becomes all the more critical for the coach (and other members of the athlete's team) to provide a sense of consistency and familiarity.

Whatever the constraints and intrusions, as coaches and practitioners we must strive to maintain the normal preparation process and competition routine as far as possible. Likewise, it is critical to remain consistent in our interactions with the athlete. This can provide a much needed sense of stability and a source of comfort for the athlete.

"Some coaches are not good competition coaches. Athletes can see fear or anger or ego, so being real, being a humanist – being what you are day in and day out in practice to me is the best recipe for success there.

— Dan Pfaff

MANAGING MINDSET...

A key role of the coach when preparing for a major competition is helping to guide how the athlete perceives the situation, where they direct their attention, and how they handle the experience.

An integral part of guiding the athlete during this time therefore concerns their faculties for exercising emotional control and managing their mental resources. It is critical that these topics have been discussed long before the athlete arrives at the event, so that the conversation on key themes can continue throughout the competition preparations.

At this time it is important to acknowledge and talk about sources of distraction, anxiety triggers, and perceived external pressures and sense of obligations felt by the athlete. Once again, these discussions should commence well in advance of the start of the competition.

These conversations can prompt a wider discussion as to the athlete's deeper motivations and drives. When dealing with a perceived threat to their self-image or status, it is important to dig deeper to what the original driver was for choosing to participate in the sport. If the athlete is looking to others for validation, or if the outcome is too inextricably tied to their sense of self-worth, then this clearly becomes a very tenuous existence. Rather they must ask themselves where they find intrinsic satisfaction in the process of practice and competition and focus on these aspects.

Clearly it is also important to provide the perspective that ultimately this is not life and death. Whatever the outcome the sun will rise the following day.

PERCEIVING THREAT VERSUS OPPORTUNITY...

Whether competition is perceived as threatening or challenging is largely a matter of interpretation. Where some athletes see threat that evokes anxiety, others may view the same competition as an opportunity and cause for excitement. This gives us scope to shift an athlete's perception, and guide them to interpret pressure conditions in a more positive manner.

For instance, it has been demonstrated in the research literature that the athlete can be guided to reappraise how they perceive the sensations of heightened physiological arousal associated with a race or a big match [129]. Shifting the athlete's perspective can entirely change how they experience and respond to what are in effect identical symptoms. In this way the athlete can experience the same feelings as excitement rather than anxiety.

Perspective has the potential to reorient the athlete's interpretation of a pressure situation. With appropriate guidance we can dramatically change how they anticipate, experience and respond to the pressure of the major competition environment. Perception has the power to change the athlete's psycho-physiological state.

The investigation by Sammy and colleagues [130] was the most recent study to demonstrate that athletes can be steered to reappraise the state of heightened physiological arousal, so that their cognitive response to the pressure condition and emotional state was far more conducive to performing. Reappraising perception of arousal was even reflected in an altered blood pressure response when performing the pressure task.

Shifting the athlete's mental representation of pressure conditions and allowing them to reappraise how they perceive associated symptoms of arousal can also influence the effects observed on performance. Whilst this has not been observed in all investigations, Moore and colleagues found that participants who reappraised threat and arousal in a positive way outperformed control subjects in the pressure task studied [131].

CULTIVATING MENTAL SKILLS AND COPING STRATEGIES...

To a large degree the task of the coach is to facilitate the athlete in managing themselves. In a previous chapter we have spoken about the importance of the athlete's awareness and ability to mobilise mental resources during training. The challenge that follows is to develop the capability to do the same in the pressure environment of a major competition.

As we have seen, with appropriate guidance the athlete can alter their perception and associated cognitive processes, affecting not only their experience of events but also the emotional and physiological responses that result. Importantly this pyscho-physiological state is more conducive to directing attention and mental effort to the task [132]. Moreover it avoids the negative effects of distraction and reinvestment of conscious control that can occur with performance anxiety.

Here too our aim is to create awareness and equip the athlete with the tools to manage themselves in different and unfamiliar environments. Our objective is to cultivate positive traits and behaviours, and hone mental skills and coping strategies. Self-awareness is a critical quality that underpins much of this; the athlete must first be able to recognise their mental state and emotional responses before they can hope to manage them. Emotional control on the part of the athlete is a critical aspect not only when they come to compete but also during the period leading up to the competition and in between sessions.

COMPETITION ARENA AS CLASSROOM...

The competition arena is always rich in opportunities to learn. It follows that major competition will be the richest time of all.

It is important that the athlete's experience at their first major competition helps them to arrive at the realisation that they have a rightful place on that stage and belong in that company.

Equally it is crucial that both coach and athlete have the perspective to look beyond the competition itself. The athlete's experiences and observations will provide invaluable insights into how and where they need to become better to succeed at that level of competition; this is an important topic for the debrief and reflection following the event.

Amidst the emotion of the event, we must acknowledge that the world doesn't end once the competition is over, whatever the result. If we assume that once the competition has ended not only will life go on, but so will the athlete, our focus can switch to working to ensure the most positive and fruitful legacy effects possible.

CHARACTER-BUILDING AND 'RESILIENCE'...

In recent times resilience has become a buzz word, and some very dubious practices have been justified in the name of developing character, as if resilient athletes can be created by punishing and often pointless workouts. In actuality, there is no need to contrive conditions and activities to build 'grit'. If managed correctly the experience of preparing for and performing in the crucible of major competitions affords abundant opportunities for developing resiliency in a way that athletes are better equipped to deal with these challenges in the future.

Coaches and athlete should always be attentive to opportunities for learning and growth. The journey of an athlete will serve up an array of obstacles; they must solve problems and negotiate a variety of barriers. The athlete will often be required to overcome adversity in their career, and in doing so they are prompted to develop strategies for coping with these challenges.

The task of the coach therefore is to help the athlete take best advantage of these naturally occurring opportunities for growth. The debrief and reflection process that follows a major competition (see Appendix) is a particularly abundant time for learning; an important role of the coach during this process is to steer the athlete's attention to the most salient lessons.

Ultimately whether the athlete is able to take advantage of the learning opportunities afforded to them depends upon the level of honesty they are able to exercise. Whilst the coach can offer guidance, this is ultimately a self-directed process that the athlete must embrace and engage with on an ongoing basis.

We have spoken before about the need for the athlete to adopt a self-regulation approach and meta-learning strategies during training. The approach to major competition and the event itself should therefore simply represent an extension of this everyday process.

There are a variety of tools the athlete can equip themselves with to assist in this process, such as maintaining a training log and a diary to record input, self-talk and reflections. Engaging in regular (daily) debriefs and periodic reviews outside of the big events are likewise integral to this process.

Appendix

Template for Review Process Post Major Competition

Looking Back:

Objectively review how well you managed the following areas:

1. Pre Event Admin

   Organisation of travel, arrangements for accommodation, communication with staff/meet organisers, awareness and adherence to schedule and protocols for the event

2. Self-management during final preparations

   Nutrition (source, choices, timing), sleep, regeneration, daily maintenance, self-therapy, mental refreshment

3. Self-regulation throughout the event

   Awareness and handling of emotional state, managing psychological arousal, mental processes, regulating attention, countermeasures to handle distractions and detractors

4. Game day process

   Admin and organisation, fuelling strategy, warm up, regulation of mental and emotional state, coping with unforeseen challenges, contingency plans, call room

5. Game plan and technical execution

Objectively rate and review your support team during final preparations and the event:

1. Therapy support

2. Interaction with therapists/other support staff

3. Coaching support during pre-event preparations

4. Coaching provided at the competition

5. Communication with coach during final preparations and on 'game day'

6. Preliminary debrief following the event

Evaluating Where We Are Now (day to day process):

Are you doing everything you can? Rate yourself in the following areas: (0 - 5 scale: 0 = Zero consideration/investment; 5 = World Class)		
Investment of Mental Resources	Focus and intention each day upon arrival at training or practice	
	Attention allocated during the session (e.g. execution of each repetition)	
	Investment of mental effort during training and practice	
Managing Self	Lifestyle and 'wellness' factors (relationships, mental health, self-care)	
	Advance management to mitigate stressors (negative interactions, known sources of stress)	
	Coping strategies during stressful situations and pressure conditions	
	Self-regulation and emotional control	
Personal Admin	Consistent attendance and compliance	
	Organisation, scheduling, managing commitments	
	Contingency planning	
Self-Maintenance	Sleep (consistency, duration, quality)	
	Nutrition (e.g. preparation, content, timing)	
	Therapy (including self-therapy) and regeneration	

Further comments on any of the above?:

Miscellaneous:

Looking Forwards:

What are your target events for the upcoming period?

What are the target outcomes you want to achieve over the short-, medium-, and long-term?

What Process Goals can you identify that are integral to these outcomes?

Priority: Rate the importance of achieving these outcomes and goals? (tick the relevant box – N.B. there are no wrong answers here)	
Most important thing in my life	
Of equal importance to other priority areas	
Fairly important, but other aspects of my life are more important	
Not hugely important, mainly for recreation	

What are you willing to invest?

How do you rate your readiness to entertain feedback and consider making changes suggested?

What changes do you view are necessary in the following areas?:

1. Nutrition

2. Personal admin

3. Lifestyle factors

4. Self-maintenance

5. Self-regulation and emotional control

6. Technical

7. Physical

What changes do you want to see implemented moving forwards (including personnel and process)?:

1. Training schedule
2. Training
3. Coaching
4. Therapy
5. Other support

Bibliography

1. Hodges NJ, Franks IM. Modelling coaching practice: the role of instruction and demonstration. Journal of sports sciences. 2002;20(10):793-811.

2. Newell KM, McDonald, P.V. Practice: A Search for Task Solutions. Enhancing Human Performance in Sport: New Concepts and Developments (American Academy of Physical Education Papers). Human Kinetics; 1992.

3. Araujo D, Davids K. Embodied cognition and emergent decision-making in dynamical movement systems. Junctures: The Journal for Thematic Dialogue. 2004(2).

4. Weast JA, Shockley K, Riley MA. The influence of athletic experience and kinematic information on skill-relevant affordance perception. Quarterly journal of experimental psychology. 2011;64(4):689-706.

5. van Andel S, Cole MH, Pepping GJ. A systematic review on perceptual-motor calibration to changes in action capabilities. Human movement science. 2017;51:59-71.

6. Seifert L, Button C, Davids K. Key properties of expert movement systems in sport : an ecological dynamics perspective. Sports medicine. 2013;43(3):167-78.

7. Bernstein N. The co-ordination and regulation of movements. Pergamon-Press; 1967.

8. Handford C, Davids K, Bennett S, Button C. Skill acquisition in sport: some applications of an evolving practice ecology. Journal of sports sciences. 1997;15(6):621-40.

9. Abrahamson D, Sánchez–García R, Smyth C. Metaphors are projected constraints on action: An ecological dynamics view on learning across the disciplines. Singapore: International Society of the Learning Sciences; 2016.

10. Liao CM, Masters RS. Analogy learning: a means to implicit motor learning. Journal of sports sciences. 2001;19(5):307-19.

11. Post PG, Aiken CA, Laughlin DD, Fairbrother JT. Self-control over combined video feedback and modeling facilitates motor learning. Human movement science. 2016;47:49-59.

12. Millar S-K, Oldham ARH, Renshaw I, Hopkins WG. Athlete and coach agreement: Identifying successful performance. International Journal of Sports Science & Coaching. 2017;12(6):807-13.

13. McGuigan MM. Extreme Positions in Sport Science and the Importance of Context: It Depends? Int J Sports Physiol Perform. 2016;11(7):841.

14. Rovelli C. Reality is not what it seems: The journey to quantum gravity. Penguin; 2017.

15. Willingham DT. Critical Thinking: Why Is It So Hard to Teach? Arts Education Policy Review. 2008;109(4):21-32.

16. Kruger J, Dunning D. Unskilled and unaware of it: how difficulties in recognizing one's own incompetence lead to inflated self-assessments. Journal of personality and social psychology. 1999;77(6):1121-34.

17. Gamble P. Comprehensive Strength and Conditioning: Physical Preparation for Sports Performance. CreateSpace Independent Publishing Platform; 2015.

18. Kim YH, Chiu CY, Bregant J. Unskilled and Don't Want to Be Aware of It: The Effect of Self-Relevance on the Unskilled and Unaware Phenomenon. PloS one. 2015;10(6):e0130309.

19. Bowes I, Jones RL. Working at the edge of chaos: Understanding coaching as a complex, interpersonal system. Sport Psychol. 2006;20(2):235-45.

20. Cormie P, McGuigan MR, Newton RU. Developing maximal neuromuscular power: part 2 - training considerations for improving maximal power production. Sports medicine. 2011;41(2):125-46.

21. Harris GR, Stone MH, O'Bryant HS, Proulx CM, Johnson RL. Short-term performance effects of high power, high force, or combined weight-training methods. J Strength Cond Res. 2000;14(1):14-20.

22. Herman DC, Onate JA, Weinhold PS, Guskiewicz KM, Garrett WE, Yu B et al. The effects of feedback with and without strength training on lower extremity biomechanics. The American journal of sports medicine. 2009;37(7):1301-8.

23. Herman DC, Weinhold PS, Guskiewicz KM, Garrett WE, Yu B, Padua DA. The effects of strength training on the lower extremity biomechanics of female recreational athletes during a stop-jump task. The American journal of sports medicine. 2008;36(4):733-40.

24. Kiely J. Periodization paradigms in the 21st century: evidence-led or tradition-driven? Int J Sports Physiol Perform. 2012;7(3):242-50.

25. Kahneman D. Thinking, fast and slow. Macmillan; 2011.

26. Gladwell M. David and Goliath: Underdogs, misfits, and the art of battling giants. Hachette UK; 2013.

27. Bang D, Frith CD. Making better decisions in groups. Royal Society Open Science. 2017;4(8):170193.

28. Lyle MA, Valero-Cuevas FJ, Gregor RJ, Powers CM. Lower extremity dexterity is associated with agility in adolescent soccer athletes. Scandinavian journal of medicine & science in sports. 2015;25(1):81-8.

29. Gamble P. Implications and applications of training specificity for coaches and athletes. Strength Cond J. 2006;28(3):54-8.

30. Kiely J. Planning for physical performance: the individual perspective: Planning, periodization, prediction, and why the future ain't what it used to be! In: Button A, Richards H, editors. Performance Psychology. Edinburgh: Churchill Livingstone; 2011. p. 139-60.

31. Latash ML. The bliss (not the problem) of motor abundance (not redundancy). Experimental brain research. 2012;217(1):1-5.

32. Drew MK, Raysmith BP, Charlton PC. Injuries impair the chance of successful performance by sportspeople: a systematic review. British journal of sports medicine. 2017;51(16):1209-14.

33. Hagglund M, Walden M, Magnusson H, Kristenson K, Bengtsson H, Ekstrand J. Injuries affect team performance negatively in professional football: an 11-year follow-up of the UEFA Champions League injury study. British journal of sports medicine. 2013;47(12):738-42.

34. Williams S, Trewartha G, Kemp SP, Brooks JH, Fuller CW, Taylor AE et al. Time loss injuries compromise team success in Elite Rugby Union: a 7-year prospective study. British journal of sports medicine. 2016;50(11):651-6.

35. Raysmith BP, Drew MK. Performance success or failure is influenced by weeks lost to injury and illness in elite Australian track and field athletes: A 5-year prospective study. Journal of science and medicine in sport / Sports Medicine Australia. 2016;19(10):778-83.

36. Kristensen J, Franklyn-Miller A. Resistance training in musculoskeletal rehabilitation: a literature review. British journal of sports medicine. 2011:bjsports79376.

37. Malliaras P, Barton CJ, Reeves ND, Langberg H. Achilles and patellar tendinopathy loading programmes : a systematic review comparing clinical outcomes and identifying potential mechanisms for effectiveness. Sports medicine. 2013;43(4):267-86.

38. Cook JL, Purdam CR. The challenge of managing tendinopathy in competing athletes. British journal of sports medicine. 2014;48(7):506-9.

39. Gamble P. Use of load and strength training modalities for management and rehabilitation of tendinopathy. New Zealand Journal of Sports Medicine. 2016;43(1):17-23.

40. Herring SAB, J.A.; Boyajian-O'Neill, L.; Franks, R.R.; Indelicato, P.; Kibler, W.B.; Lowe, W.; Matuszak, J.; Poddar, S.; Putukian, M.; Stanton, R. . The team physician and strength and conditioning of athletes for sports: a consensus statement. Medicine and science in sports and exercise. 2015;47(2):440-5.

41. Gamble P. 'Strength and conditioning' theory and practice - a need to know. New Zealand Journal of Sports Medicine. 2015;41(1):24-7.

42. Bahr R, Krosshaug T. Understanding injury mechanisms: a key component of preventing injuries in sport. British journal of sports medicine. 2005;39(6):324-9.

43. Gamble P. Movement screening protocols: Rationale versus evidence. New Zealand Journal of Sports Medicine. 2013;40(2):83-6.

44. Malone S, Owen A, Newton M, Mendes B, Collins KD, Gabbett TJ. The acute:chonic workload ratio in relation to injury risk in professional soccer. Journal of science and medicine in sport / Sports Medicine Australia. 2017;20(6):561-5.

45. Malone S, Owen A, Mendes B, Hughes B, Collins K, Gabbett TJ. High-speed running and sprinting as an injury risk factor in soccer: Can well-developed physical qualities reduce the risk? Journal of science and medicine in sport / Sports Medicine Australia. 2017.

46. van der Does HT, Brink MS, Otter RT, Visscher C, Lemmink KA. Injury Risk Is Increased by Changes in Perceived Recovery of Team Sport Players. Clinical journal of sport medicine : official journal of the Canadian Academy of Sport Medicine. 2017;27(1):46-51.

47. Timpka T, Jacobsson J, Bargoria V, Periard JD, Racinais S, Ronsen O et al. Preparticipation predictors for championship injury and illness: cohort study at the Beijing 2015 International Association of Athletics Federations World Championships. British journal of sports medicine. 2017;51(4):271-6.

48. Glazer DD. Development and preliminary validation of the Injury-Psychological Readiness to Return to Sport (I-PRRS) scale. Journal of athletic training. 2009;44(2):185-9.

49. Grooms DR, Page SJ, Nichols-Larsen DS, Chaudhari AM, White SE, Onate JA. Neuroplasticity Associated With Anterior Cruciate Ligament Reconstruction. The Journal of orthopaedic and sports physical therapy. 2017;47(3):180-9.

50. Bien DP, Dubuque TJ. Considerations for late stage acl rehabilitation and return to sport to limit re-injury risk and maximize athletic performance. International journal of sports physical therapy. 2015;10(2):256-71.

51. Grooms D, Appelbaum G, Onate J. Neuroplasticity following anterior cruciate ligament injury: a framework for visual-motor training approaches in rehabilitation. The Journal of orthopaedic and sports physical therapy. 2015;45(5):381-93.

52. Baker J, Schorer J, Wattie N. Compromising Talent: Issues in Identifying and Selecting Talent in Sport. Quest. 2017:1-16.

53. Coyle D. The talent code: Greatness isn't born, it's grown. Random House; 2010.

54. Ericsson KA. Training history, deliberate practice and elite sports performance: an analysis in response to Tucker and Collins review--what makes champions? British journal of sports medicine. 2013;47(9):533-5.

55. Wilber RL, Pitsiladis YP. Kenyan and Ethiopian Distance Runners: What Makes Them So Good? Int J Sport Physiol. 2012;7(2):92-102.

56. Coughlan EK, Williams AM, McRobert AP, Ford PR. How experts practice: a novel test of deliberate practice theory. Journal of experimental psychology Learning, memory, and cognition. 2014;40(2):449-58.

57. Collins DJ, Macnamara A, McCarthy N. Putting the Bumps in the Rocky Road: Optimizing the Pathway to Excellence. Front Psychol. 2016;7(1482):1482.

58. Gladwell M. Outliers: The story of success. Hachette UK; 2008.

59. Ford P, De Ste Croix M, Lloyd R, Meyers R, Moosavi M, Oliver J et al. The long-term athlete development model: physiological evidence and application. Journal of sports sciences. 2011;29(4):389-402.

60. Lloyd RS, Oliver JL. The Youth Physical Development Model: A New Approach to Long-Term Athletic Development. Strength Cond J. 2012;34(3):61-72.

61. Gamble P. Metabolic Conditioning Development in Youths. In: Lloyd RS, Oliver, J.L., editor. Strength and conditioning for young athletes: science and application. Routledge; 2013.

62. Mirwald RL, Baxter-Jones AD, Bailey DA, Beunen GP. An assessment of maturity from anthropometric measurements. Medicine and science in sports and exercise. 2002;34(4):689-94.

63. Hills AP, King NA, Armstrong TP. The contribution of physical activity and sedentary behaviours to the growth and development of children and adolescents: implications for overweight and obesity. Sports medicine. 2007;37(6):533-45.

64. Gamble P. Approaching Physical Preparation for Youth Team-Sports Players. Strength Cond J. 2008;30(1):29-42.

65. Brenner JS. Overuse injuries, overtraining, and burnout in child and adolescent athletes. Pediatrics. 2007;119(6):1242-5.

66. Malina RM. Early sport specialization: roots, effectiveness, risks. Current sports medicine reports. 2010;9(6):364-71.

67. Dick F. Athlete development: Reflections on the pathway from potential to performance. New studies in athletics. 2013;28(1/2):47-54.

68. Myer GD, Jayanthi N, Difiori JP, Faigenbaum AD, Kiefer AW, Logerstedt D et al. Sport Specialization, Part I: Does Early Sports Specialization Increase Negative Outcomes and Reduce the Opportunity for Success in Young Athletes? Sports health. 2015;7(5):437-42.

69. Fajen BR, Riley MA, Turvey MT. Information, affordances, and the control of action in sport. International Journal of Sport Psychology. 2009.

70. Crow JF, Buttifant D, Kearny SG, Hrysomallis C. Low load exercises targeting the gluteal muscle group acutely enhance explosive power output in elite athletes. Journal of strength and conditioning research / National Strength & Conditioning Association. 2012;26(2):438-42.

71. Loudon JK, Reiman MP. Conservative management of femoroacetabular impingement (FAI) in the long distance runner. Physical therapy in sport : official journal of the Association of Chartered Physiotherapists in Sports Medicine. 2014;15(2):82-90.

72. Skof B, Strojnik V. The effect of two warm-up protocols on some biomechanical parameters of the neuromuscular system of middle distance runners. Journal of strength and conditioning research / National Strength & Conditioning Association. 2007;21(2):394-9.

73. Headlee DL, Leonard JL, Hart JM, Ingersoll CD, Hertel J. Fatigue of the plantar intrinsic foot muscles increases navicular drop. Journal of electromyography and kinesiology : official journal of the International Society of Electrophysiological Kinesiology. 2008;18(3):420-5.

74. Jam B. Evaluation and retraining of the intrinsic foot muscles for pain syndromes related to abnormal control of pronation. Advanced Physical Therapy Education Institute. 2006.

75. Fiolkowski P, Brunt D, Bishop M, Woo R, Horodyski M. Intrinsic pedal musculature support of the medial longitudinal arch: an electromyography study. The Journal of foot and ankle surgery : official publication of the American College of Foot and Ankle Surgeons. 2003;42(6):327-33.

76. Kelly LA, Kuitunen S, Racinais S, Cresswell AG. Recruitment of the plantar intrinsic foot muscles with increasing postural demand. Clinical biomechanics. 2012;27(1):46-51.

77. Ribeiro AP, Trombini-Souza F, Tessutti V, Rodrigues Lima F, Sacco Ide C, Joao SM. Rearfoot alignment and medial longitudinal arch configurations of runners with symptoms and histories of plantar fasciitis. Clinics (Sao Paulo, Brazil). 2011;66(6):1027-33.

78. McKeon PO, Hertel J, Bramble D, Davis I. The foot core system: a new paradigm for understanding intrinsic foot muscle function. British journal of sports medicine. 2015;49(5):290.

79. Cheung RT, Sze LK, Mok NW, Ng GY. Intrinsic foot muscle volume in experienced runners with and without chronic plantar fasciitis. Journal of science and medicine in sport / Sports Medicine Australia. 2016;19(9):713-5.

80. McKeon PO, Fourchet F. Freeing the foot: integrating the foot core system into rehabilitation for lower extremity injuries. Clinics in sports medicine. 2015;34(2):347-61.

81. Morin JB, Slawinski J, Dorel S, de Villareal ES, Couturier A, Samozino P et al. Acceleration capability in elite sprinters and ground impulse: Push more, brake less? Journal of biomechanics. 2015;48(12):3149-54.

82. Morin JB, Edouard P, Samozino P. Technical ability of force application as a determinant factor of sprint performance. Medicine and science in sports and exercise. 2011;43(9):1680-8.

83. Mulligan EP, Cook PG. Effect of plantar intrinsic muscle training on medial longitudinal arch morphology and dynamic function. Manual therapy. 2013;18(5):425-30.

84. Goldmann JP, Sanno M, Willwacher S, Heinrich K, Bruggemann GP. The potential of toe flexor muscles to enhance performance. Journal of sports sciences. 2013;31(4):424-33.

85. Tam N, Tucker R, Astephen Wilson JL. Individual Responses to a Barefoot Running Program: Insight Into Risk of Injury. The American journal of sports medicine. 2016;44(3):777-84.

86. Gamble P. An integrated approach to training core stability. Strength Cond J. 2007;29(1):58-68.

87. Abe T, Tayashiki K, Nakatani M, Watanabe H. Relationships of ultrasound measures of intrinsic foot muscle cross-sectional area and muscle volume with maximum toe flexor muscle strength and physical performance in young adults. J Phys Ther Sci. 2016;28(1):14-9.

88. Willems TM, Witvrouw E, De Cock A, De Clercq D. Gait-related risk factors for exercise-related lower-leg pain during shod running. Medicine and science in sports and exercise. 2007;39(2):330-9.

89. Bandholm T, Boysen L, Haugaard S, Zebis MK, Bencke J. Foot medial longitudinal-arch deformation during quiet standing and gait in subjects with medial tibial stress syndrome. The Journal of foot and ankle surgery : official publication of the American College of Foot and Ankle Surgeons. 2008;47(2):89-95.

90. Gooding TM, Feger MA, Hart JM, Hertel J. Intrinsic Foot Muscle Activation During Specific Exercises: A T2 Time Magnetic Resonance Imaging Study. Journal of athletic training. 2016;51(8):644-50.

91. Goldmann JP, Bruggemann GP. The potential of human toe flexor muscles to produce force. Journal of anatomy. 2012;221(2):187-94.

92. Ives JC, Shelley GA. Psychophysics in functional strength and power training: review and implementation framework. Journal of strength and conditioning research / National Strength & Conditioning Association. 2003;17(1):177-86.

93. Wulf G. Attentional focus and motor learning: a review of 15 years. International Review of Sport and Exercise Psychology. 2013;6(1):77-104.

94. Behm DG, Sale DG. Intended Rather Than Actual Movement Velocity Determines Velocity-Specific Training Response. J Appl Physiol. 1993;74(1):359-68.

95. Behm DG. Neuromuscular implications and applications of resistance training. The Journal of Strength & Conditioning Research. 1995;9(4):264-74.

96. Winkelman NC. Attentional Focus and Cueing for Speed Development. Strength Cond J. 2016;Publish Ahead of Print:1.

97. Weiss SM, Reber AS, Owen DR. The locus of focus: the effect of switching from a preferred to a non-preferred focus of attention. Journal of sports sciences. 2008;26(10):1049-57.

98. Winkelman NC, Clark KP, Ryan LJ. Experience level influences the effect of attentional focus on sprint performance. Human movement science. 2017;52:84-95.

99. Perkins-Ceccato N, Passmore SR, Lee TD. Effects of focus of attention depend on golfers' skill. Journal of sports sciences. 2003;21(8):593-600.

100. Schücker L, Schmeing L, Hagemann N. "Look around while running!" Attentional focus effects in inexperienced runners. Psychology of Sport and Exercise. 2016;27:205-12.

101. Schucker L, Knopf C, Strauss B, Hagemann N. An internal focus of attention is not always as bad as its reputation: how specific aspects of internally focused attention do not hinder running efficiency. Journal of sport & exercise psychology. 2014;36(3):233-43.

102. Pelleck V, Passmore SR. Location versus task relevance: The impact of differing internal focus of attention instructions on motor performance. Acta psychologica. 2017;176:23-31.

103. Rienhoff R, Fischer L, Strauss B, Baker J, Schorer J. Focus of attention influences quiet-eye behavior: An exploratory investigation of different skill levels in female basketball players. Sport, Exercise, and Performance Psychology. 2015;4(1):62-74.

104. Querfurth S, Schucker L, de Lussanet MH, Zentgraf K. An Internal Focus Leads to Longer Quiet Eye Durations in Novice Dart Players. Front Psychol. 2016;7(633):633.

105. Toner J, Moran A. Enhancing performance proficiency at the expert level: Considering the role of 'somaesthetic awareness'. Psychology of Sport and Exercise. 2015;16:110-7.

106. Maurer H, Munzert J. Influence of attentional focus on skilled motor performance: performance decrement under unfamiliar focus conditions. Human movement science. 2013;32(4):730-40.

107. Jackson RC, Ashford KJ, Norsworthy G. Attentional focus, dispositional reinvestment, and skilled motor performance under pressure. Journal of sport & exercise psychology. 2006;28(1):49-68.

108. Schucker L, Hagemann N, Strauss B. Attentional processes and choking under pressure. Perceptual and motor skills. 2013;116(2):671-89.

109. Dimitroff SJ, Kardan O, Necka EA, Decety J, Berman MG, Norman GJ. Physiological dynamics of stress contagion. Scientific Reports. 2017;7(1):6168.

110. Kaspar K, Konig P. Emotions and personality traits as high-level factors in visual attention: a review. Front Hum Neurosci. 2012;6(321):321.

111. Zadra JR, Clore GL. Emotion and Perception: The Role of Affective Information. Wiley Interdiscip Rev Cogn Sci. 2011;2(6):676-85.

112. Jefferies LN, Smilek D, Eich E, Enns JT. Emotional valence and arousal interact in attentional control. Psychological science. 2008;19(3):290-5.

113. Bleil ME, Gianaros PJ, Jennings JR, Flory JD, Manuck SB. Trait negative affect: toward an integrated model of understanding psychological risk for impairment in cardiac autonomic function. Psychosomatic medicine. 2008;70(3):328-37.

114. Shang J, Fu Q, Dienes Z, Shao C, Fu X. Negative affect reduces performance in implicit sequence learning. PloS one. 2013;8(1):e54693.

115. Stults-Kolehmainen MA, Bartholomew JB, Sinha R. Chronic psychological stress impairs recovery of muscular function and somatic sensations over a 96-hour period. Journal of strength and conditioning research / National Strength & Conditioning Association. 2014;28(7):2007-17.

116. Stults-Kolehmainen MA, Bartholomew JB. Psychological stress impairs short-term muscular recovery from resistance exercise. Medicine and science in sports and exercise. 2012;44(11):2220-7.

117. Mann JB, Bryant KR, Johnstone B, Ivey PA, Sayers SP. Effect of Physical and Academic Stress on Illness and Injury in Division 1 College Football Players. Journal of strength and conditioning research / National Strength & Conditioning Association. 2016;30(1):20-5.

118. Sarkar M, Fletcher D. Psychological resilience in sport performers: a review of stressors and protective factors. Journal of sports sciences. 2014;32(15):1419-34.

119. Pena-Sarrionandia A, Mikolajczak M, Gross JJ. Integrating emotion regulation and emotional intelligence traditions: a meta-analysis. Front Psychol. 2015;6:160.

120. Spangler DP, Friedman BH. Effortful control and resiliency exhibit different patterns of cardiac autonomic control. International journal of psychophysiology : official journal of the International Organization of Psychophysiology. 2015;96(2):95-103.

121. Webb TL, Miles E, Sheeran P. Dealing with feeling: a meta-analysis of the effectiveness of strategies derived from the process model of emotion regulation. Psychological bulletin. 2012;138(4):775-808.

122. Josefsson T, Ivarsson A, Lindwall M, Gustafsson H, Stenling A, Boroy J et al. Mindfulness Mechanisms in Sports: Mediating Effects of Rumination and Emotion Regulation on Sport-Specific Coping. Mindfulness (N Y). 2017;8(5):1354-63.

123. Meggs J, Ditzfeld C, Golby J. Self-concept organisation and mental toughness in sport. Journal of sports sciences. 2014;32(2):101-9.

124. Toering TT, Elferink-Gemser MT, Jordet G, Visscher C. Self-regulation and performance level of elite and non-elite youth soccer players. Journal of sports sciences. 2009;27(14):1509-17.

125. Cleary TJ, Zimmerman BJ. Self-Regulation Differences during Athletic Practice by Experts, Non-Experts, and Novices. Journal of Applied Sport Psychology. 2001;13(2):185-206.

126. Jonker L, Elferink-Gemser MT, Visscher C. Differences in self-regulatory skills among talented athletes: the significance of competitive level and type of sport. Journal of sports sciences. 2010;28(8):901-8.

127. Baker J, Young B. 20 years later: deliberate practice and the development of expertise in sport. International Review of Sport and Exercise Psychology. 2014;7(1):135-57.

128. McCardle L, Young BW, Baker J. Self-regulated learning and expertise development in sport: current status, challenges, and future opportunities. International Review of Sport and Exercise Psychology. 2017:1-27.

129. Moore LJ, Wilson MR, Vine SJ, Coussens AH, Freeman P. Champ or chump? Challenge and threat states during pressurized competition. Journal of sport & exercise psychology. 2013;35(6):551-62.

130. Sammy N, Anstiss PA, Moore LJ, Freeman P, Wilson MR, Vine SJ. The effects of arousal reappraisal on stress responses, performance and attention. Anxiety, stress, and coping. 2017;30(6):619-29.

131. Moore LJ, Vine SJ, Wilson MR, Freeman P. Reappraising Threat: How to Optimize Performance Under Pressure. Journal of sport & exercise psychology. 2015;37(3):339-43.

132. Vine SJ, Freeman P, Moore LJ, Chandra-Ramanan R, Wilson MR. Evaluating stress as a challenge is associated with superior attentional control and motor skill performance: testing the predictions of the biopsychosocial model of challenge and threat. Journal of experimental psychology Applied. 2013;19(3):185-94.

Made in the USA
Columbia, SC
08 November 2018